RESEARCH HIGHLIGHTS IN SOCIAL WORK 19

Social Work and Health Care

RESEARCH HIGHLIGHTS IN SOCIAL WORK 19

Social Work and Health Care

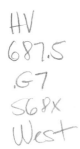

Jessica Kingsley Publishers
London

Editors: Rex Taylor and Jill Ford
Secretary: Anne Forbes
Editorial Advisory Committee:
Professor G. Rochford   University of Aberdeen
Professor J. Cheetham   University of Stirling
Dr J. Lishman   Robert Gordon's Institute of Technology
Mr S. Montgomery   Strathclyde Region Social Work Department
Mr D. Murray   Tayside Region Social Work Department (SSRG Scotland)
Dr A. Robertson   University of Edinburgh
Dr P. Seed   University of Aberdeen
Mr J. Tibbitt   Social Work Services Group, Scottish Office

University of Aberdeen
Department of Social Work
King's College
Aberdeen

First published in Great Britain in 1989 by
Jessica Kingsley Publishers Ltd
13 Brunswick Centre,
London WC1N 1AF

British Library Cataloguing in Publication Data
  Social work and health care
  1. Great Britain. Health Services. Welfare Work
  I. Taylor, Rex
  362.1'0425

ISBN 1-85302-016-8
ISSN 0955-7970

Printed in Great Britain by
Antony Rowe Ltd, Chippenham, Wiltshire

CONTENTS

Social Work and Health Care in Three Settings: 11
An Editorial Introduction
Rex Taylor and Jill Ford

Part I : The Broad Picture

Health Care and Social Work -   21
What Kind of Relationship?
Zofia Butrym

Social Work and Nursing: Sisters or Rivals?   33
Paul Bywaters

Social Work in Mental Health Teams: 47
The Local Authority Field Social Worker
Robert Brown

Anxiety and its Management in Health Care: 58
Implications for Social Work
Judith Brearley

Part II: Present Trends

Change and Diversity in Hospital Social Work   71
John Tibbitt and Ann Connor

Health Assessment of the Elderly: 89
A Multidisciplinary Perspective
Phyllis Runciman

Professional Ideology or Organisational Tribalism?   102
The Health Service-Social Work Divide
Gillian Dalley

Part III: Focus on Practice

Groupwork in General Hospitals   118
Sheila Robertson

Health Centre Social Work - Plugging the Gap?   131
A Comparative Study of Client Groups Using a
Health Centre and an Area Office
D.A. Cairns Smith

Counselling Elderly People with Mental Health Problems   152
John Carpenter

Case Recognition: 177
The Use of Vignettes in Eliciting the Social Work Response
Isobel Freeman

Contributors

Rex Taylor   Currently Professor of Social Administration and Head of Department of Social Administration and Social Work at Glasgow University. Previously MRC Research Sociologist in MRC Medical Sociology Unit and Lecturer in Sociology at Universities of Kent, Virginia (USA) and Aberdeen. Interested in community care, social work-health interface and health and social services research.

Jill Ford   After qualifying as a psychiatric social worker, Jill Ford worked for nine years in the Walthamstow Child Guidance Centre. She was also involved in community projects in Notting Hill, where she lived, and in consultancy to residential workers. In 1970 she moved to her present position as Lecturer in the Department of Social Administration and Social Work at the University of Glasgow. Here she has contributed substantially to undergraduate social administration teaching as well as to the social work programmes.

Zofia Butrym   Born in Poland. Came to England in 1947. Trained in medical social work at the London School of Economics and with the Institute of Medical Social Workers. Worked as a medical social worker at Hammersmith Hospital for eight years where latterly she also supervised students from the Carnegie Course at LSE. Was appointed as lecturer in social work at LSE in 1958. Promoted to senior lecturer in 1970. Continued to teach social work at LSE until retirement in 1987.

Paul Bywaters   Spent the 1970s qualifying as a social worker and working in Birmingham, mostly for the Social Services Department. Since 1980 has been teaching on the social work courses at Coventry Polytechnic (previously known as 'Lanchester'), apart from a brief period of research into Magistrates Domestic Courts.

Robert Brown   Principal Lecturer in social work at Croydon College. Formerly lecturer at Stirling University after seven years as student unit practice teacher (mental health) with Southampton University. Prior to that he was a social worker and then team leader with Hampshire County Council. Author of 'The Approved Social Worker's Guide to the Mental Health Act 1983' (*Community Care*). 'Money

Matters for People with a Mental Handicap' (*DIG*) and co-author of *Social Workers at Risk* (Macmillan). Recently worked in voluntary sector and consumer movement as Chairperson of Falkirk District Association for Mental Health. Continual involvement since 1982 in local authority social workers training under the new mental health legislation.

Judith Brearley   Trained in medical social work and practised in adult's and children's hospitals and in general practice. Since 1970 she has been a Lecturer in Social Work at Edinburgh University, where she teaches Human Growth and Behaviour, Residential and Day Care, and Staff Supervision in the Organisational Context. She qualified in Analytical Psychotherapy at the Scottish Institute of Human Relations, of which she is a Council Member. She has been Vice-President of SCOPE in Scotland and is Chairman of the Scottish Marriage Guidance Council. She offers consultancy to a range of organisations.

John Tibbitt   Principal Research Officer, Scottish Office, attached to Social Work Services Group. Has particular interests in links between social work and health services and methods of evaluation and performance review of Social Work Services. He has a number of publications on these topics including a study of Social Workers as Mental Health Officers and a new study, with Anne Connor, of hospital social work, to be published later this year. He is joint editor of a forthcoming volume on Performance Review in Social Work Agencies also in the *Research Highlights* series.

Anne Connor   Senior Research Officer in the Scottish Office. Joined the Civil Law Branch of the Central Research Unit in 1978 working and publishing in the fields of consumer access to the Court system and the social impact of legal processes. Moved to Social Work Services Group Branch in 1982 where her research has centred mainly on the voluntary sector and health and social work. Recent publications report findings of research on funding schemes for the voluntary sector and the work of hospital social workers.

Phyllis Runciman   Senior Lecturer - Research Development. Graduated in Social Sciences with Nursing at the University of Edinburgh. She worked in hospital and community settings as a ward sister and health visitor and carried out research related to both these fields during a nursing research training fellowship and research associate post at the University of Edinburgh. Her current work in the Department of Health and Nursing, Queen Margaret College, Edinburgh, includes developing teaching and learning strategies in relation to research and exploring research opportunities for practicing nurses.

Gillian Dalley Currently working at the King's Fund Centre for Health Services Development, London, and shortly to become a research fellow with the Centre for Health Economics, York. The research on which her contribution in this volume is based was conducted at the MRC Medical Sociology Unit, Aberdeen. She has recently written *Ideologies of Caring: Re-Thinking Community and Collectivism* (Macmillan, 1988).

Sheila Robertson Groupwork consultant. Has an M.S.W. in groupwork from the University of Pennsylvania. Initially worked in Hertfordshire as a groupwork practitioner and adviser; moved to Glasgow, and in recent years has provided groupwork consultation/training to a number of social work agencies. Taught social work at Glasgow University for two years; is now retained as a consultant by Strathclyde Social Work Department.

D.A. Cairns Smith Educated at Cheltenham Ladies College and Glasgow University. After completing a postgraduate diploma in social studies in 1963, she spent the next seven years raising her family while becoming involved in various aspects of voluntary social work. In 1978 she returned to Glasgow University to study for a CQSW where one of the electives offered was research in Social Work. After four years in an Area team in Paisley, working in a 'patch' and then with Intake and Long Term teams, she moved to Barrhead Health Centre where she undertook the research project described here. She is now in the Regional training section where she is a training supervisor of CSS students.

John Carpenter Lecturer in the Applied Psychology of Mental Health at the University of Kent at Canterbury. He graduated in psychology and qualified in social work at Bristol University and has since worked in child and adult mental health services. The project described in this volume was undertaken whilst the author held a joint appointment to the Departments of Social Work and Mental Health at Bristol University and to Avon Social Services Department (1982-87). His current interests concern the closure of long-stay psychiatric hospitals and the development of community mental health services.

Isobel Freeman   Senior Research Officer. Graduated from Strathclyde University in 1978. She undertook research into Public Attitudes to Poverty and obtained a PhD from the University of Stirling in 1984. In 1980 she joined Strathclyde Regional Council and has worked there first as research officer and later as senior research officer. Her work with the Social Work Department has involved her in research into many aspects of practice in all client groups.

Social Work and Health Care in Three Settings: An Editorial Introduction

Rex Taylor and Jill Ford

As recently as twenty-five years ago few doctors or nurses would have had any contact with anyone calling him- or herself a social worker. Those who performed a social work function did so as hospital almoners, mental welfare officers or psychiatric social workers. Times have changed, both for social workers and for health professionals. Social work has emerged as a united profession whose members share a common basic training, are employed by social work departments and mostly work in generic area teams. Those working in health settings are seconded or attached, but they remain under the ultimate control of social work departments. Over the same period, but coincidentally, demographic changes have tipped the balance of the health task from cure to care, costs of institutional care have escalated and care in the community has become both government policy and preferred professional practice.

In the light of all these developments, and particularly the pronounced swing to community care, it is paradoxical, first, that there has been no decrease in the proportion of hospital social workers, and second, that there has been no marked increase in the proportion of social workers attached to primary care teams.

Social work in hospital settings

In Scotland numbers of hospital-based social workers have increased disproportionately, and now account for one in eight of all main grade and one in four of all senior social workers (Tibbitt and Connor, chapter 5). Why have numbers continued to increase at a time when policy-makers and professionals are publicly committed to a policy of community care? One commonly offered explanation is that community care policy remains essentially rhetorical while the power of hospital consultants remains essentially real. Despite their earlier fears of losing control, hospital-based medical staff have succeeded in retaining and even increasing the numbers of seconded social workers. But this is only a partial explanation. One of the most dramatic changes in hospital work over the last fifteen years has been the increase in turnover rates. In 1971 the national average length of stay for medical patients was 14.7 days, in 1985 it was 8.7. There have been similar reductions in average lengths of stay of surgical patients and maternities. This reduction may only have been possible because of attached hospital social workers.

A link between hospital turnover rates and social worker attachments was first identified in Brandon's study[1] which compared doctors' expectations and use of social workers in three hospitals. He found a direct relationship between social worker presence and patient turnover, namely the greater the use of social workers the greater the turnover. Since then the value of a social work presence has increased as costs of patient stay have escalated. In what must be the definitive work on hospital social work yet published, Tibbitt and Connor[2] provide an illustrative account of the potential savings. They cite the example of a geriatric hospital which had 523 admissions over the course of a year and an average length of patient stay of 138 days, at a cost of £36 per day. Assuming that the introduction of on site hospital social workers would achieve a reduction of five per cent in the average length of stay, they calculated that the yearly savings would be around £130,000 per annum. Of course, set against these overall savings are the costs of the social work service and of alternative provision for patients no longer in hospital. They calculated that these costs amounted to £20,000 and £78,000 respectively, leaving net savings of £33,346 per annum. On the basis of such savings, and their estimate of a five per cent reduction in the average length of stay was cautiously modest, the case for hospital social work is already strong. On the basis of other data, including clients' views, Tibbitt and Connor identify further strengths. When the social work service was located in the hospital, rather than in an area team, it led to more effective use of the social worker's time, was better suited to the needs of clients and their families, and it enabled other hospital staff to carry out their work more efficiently and effectively.

Social work in health centres

There has been no commensurate increase in the proportion of social workers attached to health centres and primary care teams. Despite the early recommendation of one social worker per 10,000 GP population, social worker attachment to primary care units remain disappointingly low. At the beginning of the 1980s there were only twent-five social workers based in health centres in Scotland; in 1987 there were still less than forty, i.e. under two per cent of all social workers in the country. This slow, almost imperceptible growth in social worker attachment to primary care

teams is bound up with the private contractor status of GPs, but it also reflects inherent difficulties in the relationship between GPs and social workers. Huntington[3]
has mapped the terrain but it is Jeffreys and Sachs[4] who provide the most insightful
account. Their twelve year study of the Avebury and Barr practices, already a classic in the literature on general practice, deserves to be better known by social workers - as the following resumé indicates.

The Avebury and Barr practices occupy the same health centre in a densely popu-
lated area of London. The Avebury practice, established in 1953, consisted of six
GPs, two nurses, two health visitors and an attached social worker. The senior partner described himself as a 'political animal' and the practice as egalitarian. He had
pioneered social worker attachment by persuading a charitable trust to pay the sa-
lary of a social worker for an experimental period. This was deemed to have been a
success and the Avebury doctors applied to the local authority for a seconded social
worker. At the time the study started, Margaret Darby had just been appointed as
the seconded worker, half time at the Avebury and half time at the Barr practices.
The Barr practice, which had not actively campaigned for a social work attachment,
consisted of seven GPs, three attached nurses and four health visitors. It took the
name of the doctor who had founded it eighty-five years ago and most of the partners still held fairly traditional views. The senior partner was ultimately in charge
but each doctor was autonomous and had *de facto* as well as *de jure* authority over
non-medically qualified members of the team. Although attached to the two practices Margaret Darby felt herself to be 'more of an Avebury than a Barr person'.
This was mainly because of the way the two practices viewed her role and related to
her. At the Avebury practice, where the role was already established, the doctors
referred patients for her opinion, practical help, treatment and referral to other
agencies. At the Barr practice she received fewer referrals, and those she did receive
were for long-term support. There were also differences in her status in the two practices. Avebury doctors viewed her as a colleague, with skills different from, but equal
to their own. At the Barr practice she described her position as 'nebulous'. However
as a singleton (in both practices) she soon began to feel professionally isolated. The
feeling increased and she left to join an area team.

She was replaced by two workers, each working part-time in area teams. This decision to replace one full-time with two part-time workers was partly made as a result of Margaret Darby's experience of isolation. Joan Audrey, who joined the
Avebury practice, found it much to her liking. She enjoyed the high level of referral
and the predominance of short-term work, but most of all, she liked the democratic
practice ambience. Mary Bencroft, who replaced Margaret Darby at the Barr practice, was less satisfied. She had accepted the job because she had wanted to 'fly the
flag' for area social workers, but after eighteen months she felt she had made little

headway. Jeffreys and Sachs summarised her position succinctly, '(while) *accepting* her the doctors at the practice also *excepted* her'. She was also unhappy about her caseload; instead of short-term work, which she preferred, she had to spend most of her time on a small number of patients who she felt should have been referred to the area team for long-term support. It was some time before she got any referrals for short term psycho-social therapy, and then only when the doctors were too hard pressed to deal with these cases themselves. Some were clearly reluctant to refer to the social worker.

It will be apparent that while the study is of two practices only, it illustrates a number of near universal problems of social worker attachment. First, the practice philosophy and attitude of the GPs; clearly the Avebury partners were more enthusi-·astic about social work from the start. Second, the relative powerlessness of the social worker to influence the volume and nature of referrals; this was acutely felt by the social workers in the Barr practice. Third, the sense of professional isolation experienced by singleton social workers in health settings; Margaret Darby left *both* teams to return to an area office. And finally, the legitimate and understandable desire of many GPs to retain and develop their expertise in psycho-social work; Barr practice GPs viewed Mary Bancroft as a competitor for these cases.

Health care in area teams

Just how much area team social workers are currently involved in health care is difficult to determine. Following the 1983 Mental Health Act we might have expected them to be more active than hospital-based workers, simply on grounds of their greater number. Yet, as Robert Brown shows in chapter 3, this may not yet have happened. Of all the applications for detention at a Hampshire Hospital over the period 1984-1987, only eight per cent had been made by area-team workers, compared with sixty-one per cent by hospital-based social workers. Information on the current involvement of area-team social workers with other client groups is not readily available, although the impression is that it remains fairly limited. Health visitors and nurses are still more active than social workers in the care of the elderly; and despite the statutory duty on social work departments to compile disability registers, occupational therapists are more active in the care of the mentally and physically disabled. But this situation is likely to change. The National Association of Health Authorities has recently noted that while the need for social work has broadened to include support for community care, 'social work has not been able to keep pace with developments in the health services'. These developments - principally the earlier discharge of patients and the wholesale decanting of hospitals - put considerable pressure on field social work which is likely to be drawn increasingly into the health arena.

The Inter-County Workshop on Social Work Training in Health Care[5] has recently performed a valuable service in canvassing views of fieldwork teachers on coverage of health issues at the qualifying level. A questionnaire was given to a sample of fieldwork teachers (in field and health settings) and they were asked to rate the importance of a list of health topics. The major finding, summarised in Table 1, was the high level of agreement on those topics considered to be an essential component of mainstream social work readings for all social workers, regardless of the setting in which they eventually work.

As Olive Stevenson says in her preface to the report,

'the responses to the health questionnaire do not suggest that health can be relegated to a specialist corner ... a sound understanding of health-related problems is fundamental to practice in the community.'

In the last two years the Social Services Parliamentary Select Committee, the Audit Commission and Sir Roy Griffiths have all submitted reports on the future development of community care. Even if only half of their combined recommendations are eventually implemented, the implications for social work are likely to be far reaching. Griffiths has put it bluntly (perhaps too bluntly for ministerial taste):

' ... community care is a poor relation; everybody's distant relative but nobody's baby.'

His major recommendations are well known: a greater strategic role for central government, a Minister for Community Care, a more facilitative and enabling role for social work departments and new methods of financing. As far as social workers are concerned, their tasks will be to assess aggregate care needs, to identify those individuals needing care, and - taking full account of personal preferences - to offer them flexible 'packages of care'. Throughout, they will be responsible for monitoring the effectiveness and efficiency of all community care provision - including that provided by the private sector.

Social Care planning involves a focus on individuals in need rather than services, it calls for improved measures and procedures of assessment and for better measurement and monitoring of effectiveness and efficiency. Bleddyn Davies and David Challis of the Personal Social Services Research Unit at the University of Kent and Adrian Webb and Gerard Wistow at the University of Loughborough have pioneered work in this field. In Scotland the Social Work Research Centre at Stirling University is beginning to produce comparable work. Outside these centres there is

Table 1

Percentage/number of fieldwork teachers scoring topic as essential for all students

Topics	F/T in health settings	F/T in area* teams
Loss and change	76.4	12/16
Stress	73.2	10/16
The elderly	67.7	11/16
Relation of health to social class	62.2	9/16
Community care	60.6	9/16
Ethics	56.7	9/16
Alcohol and drug abuse	56.7	9/16
Psychiatric disorders	52.0	9/16
Suicide	52.0	6/16
Disability and impairment	48.8	8/16
Health care of children	44.8	10/16
Working in a multi-disciplinary team	44.1	8/16
Sexually transmitted diseases and AIDS	43.3	5/16
Normal and pathological reactions to illness	35.4	8/16
Women's health	24.4	6/16
Disease states, causes and implications	16.5	6/16
NHS - structure and development	22.8	3/16
Medical terminology and abbreviations	1.6	0/16

numbers too small to calculate percentages.

some useful work which deserves to be more widely disseminated; but overall, there is an urgent need for good evaluative research.

Of the eleven chapters in this volume, we start with that of Zofia Butrym who looks back and, in the light of this retrospective look and current developments, speculates on future trends. Her chapter, 'Health Care and Social Work - What Kind of Relationship?' focuses on the relationship between social work and medicine and uses her considerable knowledge and experience to 'philosophise' about possibilities. She is not always optimistic, unsurprisingly in these hard times perhaps, but suggests that, with a shared commitment to the improvement of services, there is hope for the future. In this 'Part I: The Broad Picture', Paul Bywaters follows by looking instead at the possible value and implications of forming an alliance between social work and nursing. In his chapter, 'Social Work and Nursing: Sisters or Rivals?', he examines this relatively unexplored area in the light of his perception that equal partnerships between social workers and doctors are unlikely to be sustainable. Also looking at social work/health care relationships is Robert Brown who focuses on multi-disciplinary work, particularly in the light of recent legislative changes, when the social worker is based in the local authority area team. In 'Social Work in Mental Health Teams: The Local Authority Field Social Worker', he considers some of the organisational issues as well as those at field level. Finally in this opening section, Judith Brearley includes collaborative and team work as one important dimension in her consideration of the all-pervasive phenomenon of anxiety and its management or mismanagement in health care settings. She focuses her study on hospital work in 'Anxiety and its Management in Health Care: Implications for Social Work'.

'Part II: Present Trends' also takes a broad approach but considers the writers' own recent research when considering present trends in particular areas of work. John Tibbitt and Ann Connor, in 'Change and Diversity in Social Work', look not only at the variable nature of hospital social work but also at instances where hospital based social work involvement offers a better service to clients and reduces time in hospital. Phyllis Runciman, although less specifically focused on social work, looks at the perspectives and assumptions of a number of different professionals when assessing need in her chapter, 'Health Assessment of the Elderly at Home: A Multi-Disciplinary Perspective'. Gillian Dalley also considers the assumptions of different professional groups, both about themselves and each other, this time in relation to wider policy issues. In 'Professional Ideology or Organisational Tribalism? The Health Service-Social Work Divide', she also notices times when there is more in common across professional boundaries but at a similar organisational level - more in common between managers, for example, whatever their profession.

'Part III: Focus on Practice', as its title suggests, considers instances of carefully monitored practice. Some monitoring, such as Sheila Robertson's 'Groupwork in General Hospitals', consists of careful recording and thoughtful evaluation; whereas others, namely D. A. Cairns-Smith's 'Health Centre Social Work - Plugging the Gap?' and John Carpenter's 'Counselling Elderly People with Mental Health Problems' include a more systematised recording system. The first shows how a single worker can introduce a monitoring system which is not too unwieldy and allows for interesting comparisons between, for example, referrals to area teams and to health centres; the second is a more elaborately developed project, itself designed in response to the findings of a previous research study, offering a specific service with evaluative research built in from the outset. Finally Isobel Freeman, in 'The Recognition of the Mental Health Aspects of Social Work Cases', illustrates an interesting way of assessing the likely response of social workers, both individually and as a member of an area team, to work involving health (in this instance mental health) problems.

This volume, then, sets the scene with a review of the current state of social work and health care informed by knowledge and experience and presented from different perspectives. It looks particularly at the relationship between the two and sets developments both in their historical and current political contexts. Also, in Brearley's chapter, the broader picture is skillfully woven with the very personal impact of pain and anxiety and the interaction of these two elements is explored in terms both of personal caring and policy development; the 'private troubles and public issues' of C. Wright Mills. This is followed by the use of recent, hitherto unpublished, research to identify (sometimes surprisingly) and illuminate current trends in hospital, primary care and wider community/policy dimensions. Finally, in its examination of practice effectiveness and possible improvements, the final *raison d'etre* of the whole enterprise is addressed - the usefulness for actual and potential consumers of the service. All chapters include interesting reflection, in the light of the findings or observations presented, on possible implications for future trends and developments.

There are, however, many different aspects of health care and of social work practice referred to and described in this volume and readers may find other types of organisation more congenial to their interests. For example, the three settings identified above are looked at by different writers: hospitals by Tibbitt and Connor, Robertson and Brearley; primary care settings by Runciman, Dalley, Cairns-Smith and Carpenter; community care by Brown and Freeman. The question of collaboration, co-operation, multi-disciplinary and team work is discussed in different contexts in a number of chapters: in general terms by Dalley and Runciman; in community care by Brown; between social workers and doctors by Butrym and between social workers and nurses by Bywaters; in relation to the management of anxiety by Brearley. Different social work practice approaches are investigated: Carpenter describes the use of counselling in work with elderly people at risk; Robertson looks at group work with hospitalised patients; Brown considers elements of community development and community care; Cairns-Smith and Freeman both investigate generic work with individuals and families. Historical development and influence is traced and considered by both Butrym and Tibbitt.

Having outlined, albeit briefly, the value of this volume, it must, however, be said that there are inevitably some concerns which receive less attention than their importance deserves. There are many specific illnesses, conditions and syndromes where developments create new possibilities (and all too frequently new problems) for diagnosis and treatment. In others, most dramatically AIDS, changing incidence or recognition create epidemic conditions with repercussions far beyond social and health care workers. Although a number of chapters consider these questions, they are not given the higher profile of separate chapters. There is some concentration, however, on specific conditions: Brown and Freeman concentrate on the field of mental health and illness; Runciman and Carpenter on work with the elderly; Robertson on work with amputees, people with head injuries and with pre-menstrual conditions; she and Brown also look at the needs of relatives. It is also arguable that too little space is given to the inequalities observable in health care provision and usage, outlined so persuasively in the Black Report and, of course, crucial to much of the social work/health interface. Butrym, Tibbitt, Cairns-Smith and Brown, however, do include consideration of inequality and inadequacy as they relate to poverty and ethnic minority groupings in this country (Cairns-Smith noting, for example, that in a whole year of work only one person who saw her was in receipt of their full benefit entitlement). Neither is the consumer viewpoint given a specific chapter but again a number of references are to be found - in Brown, Brearley, Tibbitt, Butrym and Cairns-Smith in particular. It is worth contemplating a future edition of *Research Highlights* which would address the issue of consumer evaluation in relation to the social work/health care dimension and include the views of those at the 'unequal' end of the receipt of services, as identified in the Black Report and elsewhere.

In the meantime, however, there is much of value in this volume which can be enjoyed in its own right as well as being, we hope, a prelude to future editions.

References

1. Brandon, J., 'Functions of hospital based social workers.' *Social Work Today* 1970 Vol. 1 No. 3

2. Tibbett, J., and Connor, A. *Social Workers and Health Care in Hospitals.* HMSO, 1988

3. Huntington, J. *Social Work and General Practice Medicine*. London: Allen and Unwin, 1981

4. Jeffrys, M. and Sachs, H. *Rethinking General Practice*. London: Tavistock, 1983

5. Mark, S. *The Training Needs of Social Workers in Health Care*. Oxford: Inter-County Workshop. Mimeo, 1987

Health Care and Social Work
- What Kind of Relationship?

Zofia Butrym

Consideration of this complex subject is made more difficult by a number of ambiguities and disagreements surrounding the nature of both health care and social work.

Health care*

Following the many scientific and technological developments which have taken place since the Renaissance and as a result of the growth in popularity of scientism in philosophical thought derived from these achievements, the model of health care which became prominent early this century was the organic (or mechanistic) one. This model is based on the view that the human body is analogous to a complex machine in which malfunctioning parts can be repaired or replaced and health thus restored. It provides little scope for an interest in or commitment to specifically human aspects of functioning such as the effects of subjective experience resulting from social and environmental factors, or of inner states such as anxiety, resentment, insecurity and motivation.

Medical attitudes towards pain provide a good example of the effects of an exclusively scientific outlook. The perception of pain as a purely neurological phenomenon has led many doctors to deny the reality of pain for which no physiological cause can be found. In addition to this resulting in much pain being ignored regardless of the effects of such a denial on the 'pain bearers', it also meant that the only treatments recognised for pain were those of a physical or chemical nature, i.e. surgical intervention or drugs.

---

* *The omission in this article of any reference to nurses and other health personnel is deliberate in order to simplify the discussion and does not imply a lack of recognition of their crucial importance in health care.*

Failure to incorporate into medical thought and practice insights from the humanities has led to many practices which are now, in retrospect, recognised as having been insensitive as well as uninformed. The treatment of young children in hospitals is one example of this. Separation from their parents by severe restriction on visiting was justified by its supposedly preventing upset! Another manifestation of the failings of scientism in the approach to sick people was the extent of the denial of their right to knowledge and involvement in decision making about their own bodies. 'Carrying patients in ignorance'[1] was not only widely practised but often regarded as a virtue.

In recent times, especially since World War II, the contribution of the behavioural and social sciences has led to an extended view of health and disease as being products of complex and interacting factors in the realm of biology, psychology, spirituality and environment, both human and material. Such changes in health care as the admission to hospital of parents with their children, the hospice movement and the growing respectability of psychosomatic medicine, are reflections of the effects of this enhanced understanding. What is very striking however is the reluctance and the slowness with which the new knowledge and insights are being incorporated into main stream medical practice. Most people's experience of their consultations with doctors still reflects a surprising lack of interest in them as individual people whose health problems are closely interwoven in terms of both cause and effect into their total life experience. The continuing narrow concentration in medicine on the physiological aspects at the expense of a more holistic approach is not confined to practice in highly scientific and specialised centres such as teaching hospitals. It is equally widespread in general practice in spite of numerous findings that a very large proportion of the problems brought to general practitioners is of an existential nature.

How can we explain this striking discrepancy between on the one hand the existence of relevant and useful knowledge and on the other the failure to use that knowledge by a profession committed to informed practice?

At the risk of oversimplifying what is obviously a complex phenomenon, we can nevertheless refer to a few relevant factors.

One of these is the powerful and seductive nature of positivism which causes people to view with suspicion all knowledge which is not subject to 'scientific' validation. It is hardly surprising therefore that within a positivist culture the results of an X-ray or a laboratory test are automatically granted a higher status and more credibility than a patient's subjective account of his symptoms and his/her own reflections on their possible causation.

Closely linked to the factor of the 'respectability' of scientifically validated knowledge is the attractiveness of that knowledge in terms of its clearly delineating and limiting the area of medical concern. This has a dual advantage: it makes the doctor's job more manageable and it also invests him with expertise of a distinct and exclusive kind.

In contrast, a more holistic orientation exposes the doctor to all the uncertainties which accompany the realm of knowledge concerning man as a unique ontological entity and as a social being. He can no longer feel so confident in relation to his 'material' or claim an exclusive expertise. On the contrary, in order to marshal and use constructively this vast and potentially relevant knowledge he is dependent on the help of others. Such a multi-disciplinary approach calls for a very different orientation from that based on an exclusive expertise and the temptation to omnipotence derived from it. It can make the doctor's job feel more complicated and diffuse. It can also be experienced as a threat to his status: membership of a team implies the acceptance of interdependence. In the light of these factors it is not altogether surprising that so many doctors are so reluctant to incorporate into their practice even the most elementary insights from such fields of study as anthropology, psychology, sociology and religion.

Social work

The problems of identity in social work have been fully discussed elsewhere[2] but a few historical reflections are necessary in order to place the current dilemmas in context.

The developments following from the Kilbrandon[3] and the Seebohm[4] Reports have been a turning point for contemporary social work in terms of both positive developments such as an enhanced role in society and the negative effects of loss of cohesion and dilution of professionalism. Both reports were primarily concerned with the reorganisation of local authority social services and both have recommended the creation of unified departments.

Given the range of functions these departments were expected to carry and the divergent needs of their clientele, it would seem an undisputed fact that they had to be multi-disciplinary if they were to be effective in carrying out their mandate. In view of this obvious reality it is surprising that more attention was not given at the outset to a task analysis in order to find the most appropriate and effective use of the different resources. The lack of such an analysis has led to a tendency to equate all the tasks of the new departments with social work (their name of 'Social Work Departments' in Scotland did not help matters in this respect) and to the absence of a clear vision of the particular contribution social workers can make in partnership with others. This, coupled with the parallel confusion between 'generic departments' and 'generic social work' made social work practice increasingly prone to a dilution of knowledge and skills and a resulting loss of a sense of direction.

How did such a state of affairs come about and who is to blame? An attempt to answer these questions is necessary for the purpose of delineating possible future directions.

In the light of the far reaching consequences of their recommendations it is surprising that neither the Kilbrandon nor the Seebohm Report concerned itself more specifically with the means of implementation of their proposals. However attractive the highly idealistic stance adopted in these reports, it could hardly be considered adequate in the light of the radical nature of the proposals for organisational change. As already suggested, the failure to distinguish between social services in general and social work as one particular form of social service, was a major failing.

This lack of differentiation of function was further compounded by the administrative practices in the new departments. Thus it was not uncommon to find both qualified social workers and welfare assistants carrying the same kinds of caseloads with the inevitable result that a considerable proportion of both these workers' clients failed to receive the service they required.

Failure to recognise the key importance of managerial functions and the need to provide appropriate training to senior social workers to undertake these, was another common omission. Many of the policies with regard to the deployment of social workers in the new departments, including the expectation concerning 'generic' work, reflected a lack of understanding by administrators and others of the nature of social work and in particular of the conditions necessary in order for its practice to reflect expertise and competence.

What part did social workers themselves play in creating these problems? However tempting this might be, it would be mistaken to underestimate their contribution.

Most social workers greeted the recommendations of the Kilbrandon and Seebohm Reports with uncritical enthusiasm. This was largely due to the increasing frustration experienced by many of them in respect of their role and tasks under the existing structures. Following World War II social work underwent many changes which resulted in its becoming a much more sophisticated and united profession, conscious of the contribution it was capable of making to the wellbeing of society. The constraints imposed by the existing agencies within which they operated made many social workers view practice in the so-called 'secondary settings' as being unnecessarily handicapping and they longed for a setting of their own. The newly created departments following the Kilbrandon and Seebohm Reports seemed an answer to this prayer.

It was probably the combination of this unquestioning enthusiasm and the lack of a sufficiently strong professional identity (the British Association of Social Workers was coming into being at the same time as the new departments were being set up) which made social workers opt out of their responsibility to be selective over the roles and tasks they were prepared to undertake in order to ensure that they could carry them out completely. An additional problem at the time derived from a confusion over values which was prevalent among social workers in the 1970s. This led to an equation of equality with uniformity and consequently caused a reluctance on the part of many to take part in any form of differentiation of roles and tasks, this being interpreted as elitism. Thus, for social workers to delegate tasks to welfare assistants and use them for the carrying out of more straightforward work was seen to be denigrating. Equally, specialisation and any claims to particular expertise, were apt to be viewed with suspicion and disapproval for reasons of political ideology rather than to be judged by professional criteria.

Whatever the reasons, the effects of the diffusion of the roles of local authority social workers led to an increasing lack of public confidence in them and a consequent readiness by the public media to scapegoat them. One particularly serious result of this poor public image was the obstacle it created to constructive working partnerships between social workers and members of the other helping professions, doctors included.

The setting up of the Barclay Committee on the role and functions of social workers in local authority Social Services Departments was an attempt to understand the problems facing local authority based social work and to suggest remedies. However, the Report of the Committee[5], apart from acknowledging the importance and worth of social workers' contribution as well as the difficulties of their task, did little to elucidate the latter or make it more manageable. Rather, on the contrary, in keeping with some of the less desirable academic propensities of social work it proceeded to reformulate a few of the key concepts of social work instead of attempting to clarify their application in the social services department setting. Examples of this are the substitution of 'social policing' for 'social control' and 'counselling' for 'casework'. Even more unhelpfully, it came firmly down in favour of not differentiating between social work and social services on the grounds that they are seen as indistinguishable by most people and because of the value of viewing social work as a wide ranging activity!

The cumulative effect upon social workers of the lack of clarity about their role and tasks which has increasingly meant that they could neither feel adequately equipped for the job themselves nor be in a position to defend themselves against unrealistic expectations or unfair criticism by others, has been a loss of morale and much premature 'burn out'. The combination of the extensive mandate vested in

Social Work and Social Services Departments, often not matched by adequate resources, with social workers being held predominantly responsible for its fulfilment,
has highlighted the negative aspects of the monopoly of a 'social workers' own setting' for both social workers and clients. A recognition of this fact is an important
preliminary to a discussion of the nature of the relationship between health care and
social work and of how it can be strengthened.

Health care and social work past and present

Health care and social work share a concern for the wellbeing of individuals, families
and social groups. That this concern calls for collaboration if it is to be truly effective has been recognised by some doctors and some social workers since the first
hospital almoners were placed in voluntary hospitals by the Charity Organisation
Society at the end of the last century. In spite of the relationship between the two
professions being frequently fraught with difficulties and having lacked in equality
of recognition and status, in the years following on the creation of the National
Health Service and before the 'take-over' of hospital social workers by the local
authorities in the 1970s, the place of medical social work was firmly established in
many hospitals and the service was proving highly effective in improving the quality
of patients' and their families' experience of medical treatment and care.

The fact that the achievements of the objectives of health care and of social work
are mutually dependent stems from the nature of both. A holistic orientation to
health inherently calls for a multi-disciplinary approach in which social work, with
its focus on people's psycho-social functioning, must be an essential ingredient.
Equally, a sound grasp of the bio-psycho-social unity in human life must result in social workers recognising the important part played by health as both cause and effect in problems of personal functioning.

Given the obvious nature of the inter-dependence between health care and social work some explanation is necessary of why the acceptance of this fact has been
so partial and often so half-hearted on the part of both social workers and doctors.
The reasons for the wide discrepancy in this field between logic and practice are
largely derived from a complex interaction of attitudinal, social and cultural, and
structural and organisational factors.

In the realm of attitudes, there are some powerful stereotypes held by both doctors and social workers of each other which have prevented co-operation. These
have largely to do with distorted perceptions of each other's role and functions. Thus
some social workers tend to view doctors as being more omniscient and powerful
than they really are. They contrast this supposed omnipotence with their own equally

unrealistic ignorance and powerlessness in relation to the problems they deal with. The result tends to be either an excessive awe or a powerful resentment of doctors, neither of which attitudes is conducive to a constructive partnership.

Those doctors whose commitment to scientific evidence and foolproof certainty is too exclusive can readily mistake social workers' concern with 'soft data' and the uniqueness of personal experience for a lack of intellectual rigour, indecisiveness, or even incompetence.

Included under attitudinal obstacles to collaboration must also be the failure on the part of some doctors and some social workers to adopt an adequate 'service orientation' to their work which puts the patient/client and his/her needs first. Where such an orientation is lacking such factors as personal convenience, personal dislike, professional competitiveness or jealousy, may come to the fore and prevent the sharing of knowledge and responsibility required to maximise the effects of therapeutic intervention.

Many of the attitudinal problems discussed above stem from a number of cultural and social differences between the two professions which are in turn rooted in their history. In spite of the growing recognition of the holistic nature of health, medicine, as already suggested, is still predominantly science oriented whilst the primary orientation of social work is a humanistic one. This cultural dichotomy between the two professions is further enhanced by the difference of status. Medicine is a much older profession than social work and is firmly established in society, holding a much more prestigious position. A consequence of this is that the relationship between doctors and social workers often lacks equality and the mutual trust and respect which are necessary for it to be effective.

Different professional cultures result in different priorities and emphases and these can and do result in conflict. Although modern versions of the Hippocratic oath commit doctors to practice which aims 'to cure sometimes, to alleviate often, to comfort always', in reality the focus of a scientifically oriented medicine is largely on curing with relatively little attention being devoted to the tasks concerned with the maintenance of chronic conditions or support of those who are incurably ill.

In contrast, the central area of concern of social work is that of the quality of living. Inherent in this is the recognition that physical disease is only one aspect of human life which influences its quality, and not always the most important one. Given that perspective, social workers are often more inclined than are doctors to pay attention to the effects of a treatment on a given individual and his/her life style irrespective of the treatment's 'objective' value. Where social work is practised in genuine partnership with medicine, this psycho-social orientation of the former can bring valuable insights and make a very real contribution to the diagnostic and therapeutic tasks of the latter.

In addition to the attitudinal and cultural/social impediments to an effective partnership between doctors and social workers, the current organisational structures within which the two professions operate militate strongly against such a collaboration. The current position of hospital social workers is one apt illustration of this point. Since the post-Kilbrandon and Seebohm reforms, these workers have found themselves in a highly ambiguous situation. Those who work full time in hospitals have to combine a committed membership of multi-disciplinary hospital teams with all that this entails, with the status of an employee of a local authority. Such an arrangement, creating as it does inevitable conflicts over loyalties, priorities, etc., is unsatisfactory at the best of times. Given the extent of the current difficulties facing health services and local authority social services in their relationship to each other, especially over the provision of services to such vulnerable and 'care intensive' groups as old people and those suffering from either a chronic mental disorder or severe disability, hospital social workers find themselves at the centre of conflict and are in a 'no-win' situation. They are often seen as unwelcome outsiders by both the hospital staff and their local authority colleagues and their relationships with the latter are not made any easier by the very low priority usually given to social work involvement in health care by local authority managers. This is often seen as a luxury service, a soft option and an unwarranted deployment of scarce resources. It hardly needs stating that such a climate is hardly conducive to the promotion of an imaginative and high quality practice.

A further serious obstacle to the development of expertise in medical social work has been the disavowal of specialisation within social work since the post-Kilbrandon and Seebohm developments to which reference has already been made. This has had a cumulative effect. As the supply of experienced medical social workers has been drying up as a result of retirement and promotion to managerial posts in social services departments, new entrants into hospital social work have been recruited from area team generic social workers. At first, this applied to basic grade staff only, but gradually senior social workers too entered hospitals without having had any prior experience of or specific training in social work with ill people. This has meant increasingly that even those social workers who come to work in hospitals from training courses with a particular interest in this form of social work are being deprived of expert staff supervision which would help them to develop the necessary specialist knowledge and skills.

These developments have both contributed to and have been reinforced by changes in the nature of much of hospital social work since the 1970s. This has increasingly become largely a liaison service between the hospital and the local authority social services department concerned. On the one hand it tries to ensure the prompt arrangement of the necessary social services for patients being discharged from hospital and on the other has to justify to hospital staff anxious to ensure a quick turnover of beds the non-availability of certain resources or the delay in their provision. Hospital social workers have been, of course, always involved in after-care and liaison functions of this kind: it is the present prominence and even exclusiveness of these which distorts and diminishes the potential social work contribution to health care in the hospital setting. A dual situation results in which many patients who could have benefited from a social worker's intervention are not referred and some of the less 'tangible' needs of those who have been referred for the provision of specific social services are not attended to for lack of time or commitment.

The area of primary health care is in many ways an obvious setting for social work. A number of studies including those by Goldberg and Neill[6] and Huntington[7] have shown both the need for a social work contribution to that field and the extent of the scope it offers for such involvement being truly effective, not least in stopping through secondary prevention an escalation of the problems. In spite of this evidence, meaningful attachments of social workers to general practices remain very few. The emphasis on 'meaningful' is important because it helps to differentiate between the numerous 'liaison schemes' between local authority social services departments and general practices on the one hand and the small number of full time attachments of social workers to general practices on the other. Whilst the former may serve a useful administrative function they cannot be regarded as a genuine partnership between primary health care and social work. For such a partnership to be viable the social worker must be an integral member of the general practice team and not a fleeting visitor whose primary commitment and loyalties lie elsewhere.

It is a sad reflection on both health care and social work policy makers that in spite of all the evidence pinpointing the importance of a truly holistic approach to primary health care, so little commitment has been shown so far to effecting such an approach. A good example of such failure is the recent DHSS document on primary health care[8] which contains no reference to social work at all. Social work itself must however accept a large measure of responsibility for this neglect because within its own scheme of priorities during the last twenty years an involvement in health care has been ascribed a very low place indeed.

What of the future?

If the present wide gap between the desirable and the extant with regard to the relationship between health care and social work is to be bridged major changes in both are necessary.

Doctors need to become more convinced about the claims of holistic health care and they must be both taught such care and made accountable for providing it. Given the importance of economic considerations in the present political climate evidence must be collected to demonstrate that in addition to the less tangible effects on human well being of an approach which relates to the whole person in his/her social context, such an approach is also a money saver in that it maximises the effects of any medical treatment or rehabilitation.

Social workers have an important part to play in providing such evidence, but for this to be possible they must make a stronger commitment to multi-disciplinary work in health care. This will necessitate in turn a modification of the post-Kilbrandon and post-Seebohm ideology concerning both generic social work and the local authority social services department as a setting.

The fundamental difference between 'generic' meaning 'shared' and particularly applicable to a common educational base, and 'generic' as synonymous with 'all purpose', was forcibly pinpointed by Timms.[9] This difference assumes a particular importance at the time of the present crisis in social work education. One must hope that the recent refusal by Government to provide funds for an additional third 'specialist' year will not lead to the abandonment of a common educational base for all social workers and a return to pseudo-specialisms of the past. Such a base is essential for the furthering of professional knowledge and skills and without it social work would risk becoming merely a technology. Parallel with this requirement is however the need to abandon the myth of a generic practice and to replace it with a commitment to developing appropriate specialisms following on the basic generic education and training. Without such a commitment social work cannot expect to become sufficiently competent and expert to fulfil the growing expectations of society.

Issues of professional practice cannot be considered without reference to organisational structures. In this respect a strong case can also be made out for radical changes. One of these relates to the need for social work to reconsider its position in relation to, so called, 'secondary settings'. In the light of the experience of recent years it is increasingly difficult to reconcile the service orientation inherent in social work with an exclusive commitment to the one setting of a local authority social services department. Human needs and problems are not confined to any one context and they have to be met wherever they present themselves. A further strong argument in favour of diversification in relation to setting derives from the awareness that multi-disciplinary work is a common requirement for the work of any one profession to be truly effective. This is obvious in the context of health care but is seen to be equally important in other fields.

In considering specifically the relationship between health care and social work one cannot ignore the obstacles to this relationship which are created by the current administrative structures. As has already been noted, the removal of hospital social work from the National Health Service has not been beneficial to the partnership between health care and social work. The same can be argued in relation to the broader boundaries concerning the respective responsibilities of health and social services for the care of certain vulnerable groups of clients/patients like old people. How valid is the present distinction between nursing homes which are the responsibility of the health service and old people's homes which are under the jurisdiction of local authorities? Community care provision for this and other vulnerable groups has been thwarted by the ambiguities surrounding such basic considerations as source of financial support and the nature of accountability. It is a field ripe for 'buck passing' and for mutual recriminations instead of a close partnership between the health and the social care components of the services required.

The recent report by Sir Roy Griffiths[10] which specifically addresses this issue suggests that local authority departments should take over full responsibility for community care and should draw on the health services as required. In the light of the above arguments, this recommendation, if implemented, could prove a very mixed blessing. On the positive side, if accepted, the new system would do away with the ambiguities concerning responsibility, finance and accountability and would put all these firmly in the local authority court. However, the price to be paid for such a solution could be a heavy one, in that it would not only sever the existing links between health care and social work, but it would also make an integrated and holistic approach to the needs of elderly people, people with chronic disabilities and mental disorder more difficult. At its worst, it could certainly provide an excuse for doctors to opt out of their responsibilities towards these patients or to reduce them to a minimum.

Therefore, in spite of Sir Roy's dismissal of this alternative, there is a strong argument in favour of unification of those health and social services which are concerned with such vulnerable groups, as the best way to ensure an integration of their health and social care. Reasons of size need not be an insuperable obstacle to such an organisational arrangement since administrative efficiency and viability can be achieved by the creation of appropriately localised units and by attention to consumer opinion.

A restructuring of services cannot be a substitute for a commitment to a closer collaboration on the part of all concerned, but if the case for a close integration of health care and social care is accepted, then there is a credible argument that such shared care is most likely to be achieved and to be carried out effectively within a unified organisational structure.

References

1. Statement (unpublished) by an eminent member of the Royal College of Surgeons made in the 1960s.

2. Butrym, Z.T. *The Nature of Social Work.* Macmillan, 1976.

3. G.B. Scottish Home and Health Department, Scottish Education Department. *Children and Young Persons, Scotland.* Cmnd. 2306, HMSO, 1964.

4. DHSS. *Report of the Committee on the Local Authority and Allied Personal Social Services.* Cmnd. 3703, HMSO, 1968.

5. Barclay Committee Report. *Social Workers: Their Role and Tasks,* 1982.

6. Goldberg, E.M. and Neill, J.E. *Social Work in General Practice.* Allen and Unwin, 1973.

7. Huntington, J. *Social Work and General Medical Practice: Collaboration or Conflict.* Allen and Unwin, 1981.

8. DHSS. *Primary Health Care: An Agenda for Discussion.* Cmnd. 9771, HMSO, 1986.

9. Timms, N. *The Language of Social Casework.* Routledge and Kegan Paul, 1968.

10. Griffiths, R. *Community Care: Agenda for Action: A Report to the Secretary of State for Social Services.* HMSO, 1988.

Social Work and Nursing: Sisters or Rivals?

Paul Bywaters

Introduction

For eighty years co-operation with doctors has been seen as essential to social work in 'health settings' (hospitals and primary health care teams).[1,2,3,4] There can be no question that social workers in health settings have to work with members of other occupational groups. However, there is equally little doubt that doctors have not shown a reciprocal interest in their relationships with social workers, nor have they focussed so intensely upon co-operation or collaboration as the necessary form of relationship. Moreover the reality of these relationships has been characterised more by misunderstanding and struggle than by mutual respect and equal exchange. As Parsloe has put it:

'It is fashionable to exhort doctors and social workers to co-operate...but so far as we know, exhortation is quite ineffective...it tends to obscure the complexities of co-operation in a cloud of good intentions'.[5]

In the last ten years some re-evaluation of social workers' relationships with other health workers has begun to take place.[6,7,8,9,10] Sociological analysis of inter-professional relationships (for example, Friedson,[11]) is in stark contrast to the mostly optimistic tone of social work literature. As Stacey[12] concludes:

'the division of labour within this area of health and illness is always open to conflict, negotiation and change.'

In a previous essay I questioned

'What gains have been achieved for social work or its clients by the espousal of co-operation with medicine as its first principle?'[10]

I argued that, in order to maximise its contribution to health care, social work needed to clarify the values and concepts of health and illness on which it is based, and suggested that social work in health settings was not necessarily dependent upon good relationships with doctors. Possible alternatives included creating alliances with other health workers or with 'consumers', working independently, or opposing aspects of medical domination. Here I want to pursue one of those avenues in greater detail by exploring the problems and possibilities of social work's relationship with nursing.

Oakley's paper 'On the Importance of Being a Nurse' begins with a 'personal confession of blindness to the importance of nursing'.[13] Her contrition should be shared by social work. Once realised, the lack of attention paid to the relationship between social work and nursing is even more remarkable than the amount of attention paid by social work to the medical profession.

The argument below begins by trying to establish whether there is significant common ground between social work and nursing, either in terms of occupational structure, or in the knowledge base, values, and work processes revealed in each occupation's search for professional status. I will suggest that this examination reveals more mutuality than Huntingdon demonstrated between social workers and general practitioners.[7] but that this may be as likely to lead to increased conflict over occupational 'territory' as to greater co-operation or easier working relationships. Finally I make some observations about the possibility of alliances based on values and interests which transcend occupational boundaries.

Throughout, the terms 'social worker' and 'nurse' will be used to refer primarily to qualified members of each occupation. However, in places the argument requires consideration of the position of unpaid and paid workers doing auxiliary or allied jobs to nursing or social work, at lower levels of training, qualification and remuneration. There are also distinctions to be made between social workers (or nurses) and social work (or nursing); between practitioners and the occupational group to which they belong. It is, of course, always problematic to talk about such a group as if it were a homogeneous entity.

Social work and nursing: structural similarities

Both social work and nursing are predominantly female occupations, in terms of the overall numbers of workers and their public images. Approximately 90 per cent of the nursing workforce is women, men not being admitted to the Royal College of Nursing (RCN) until 1960. However this simple general picture masks some significant variations within nursing. Whereas only about five per cent of nursing auxiliaries and assistants are male, the proportion rises to one male to ten female students, and one to five of registered nurses, while nearly half of the senior management and education jobs are occupied by men, including the post of General Secretary at the RCN.[14] There are also significant differences in the proportion of men in different areas of nursing. In 1970 nearly three-fifths of nurses working with people who were mentally ill or mentally handicapped were male.

The pattern within social work and the personal social services is similar.[15] The proportion of women is again in inverse relationship to the level of pay and power within the social services organisations. Thus in 1977 (the last year for which statistics were collected by the DHSS) three-quarters of care staff in residential homes were female, compared to three-fifths of basic grade social workers, half of team leaders, nut only eight per cent of Directors of Social Services or Chief Probation Officers. There is also a parallel division of labour within each grade. Howe's study[15] found that workers with caseloads heavily weighted towards elderly people were much more likely to be women, while social work with mentally ill and mentally handicapped people was more likely to be done by men. In this context it is interesting that almost all hospital social workers were female.

The levels of pay are also not dissimilar. Recent pay awards to nurses have placed ward sisters in a range offering broadly the same rewards as Level Three social workers and team leaders. Newly qualified nurses' pay will range from £8,000 to £10,000 p.a., close to that of level 1 and 2 qualified social workers. The pay scales have also been subject to restructuring for similar reasons, including the need to create 'career grades' to retain experienced practitioners in frontline posts.

Nurses and social workers may be described as service occupations, in the dual sense of servicing both clients and other occupations (for example, medicine or the law).[16] In each case the predominant locus of employment is in large, hierarchical organisations which employ staff in a variety of occupations. There is a contrast with the independent contractor status of many doctors. For both groups, promotion tends to result in a move away from direct contact with clients, and into a managerial relationship with other nurses or social workers, while the least qualified members have the most direct contact. Within hospitals, both are significantly affected by the legal responsibility for patients resting with Consultants, so that their roles are institutionalised as secondary. However, it can be argued that the preeminence of social work within Social Services Departments as a whole is unlike the position of nursing within the NHS.

There are several further important structural differences between the occupations. A key area is education. As Trevor Clay, the present General Secretary of the RCN, revealingly put it,

'with training based in higher education, social workers have an intellectual cache (sic), representing the cerebral against nursing's practical bent'.[17]

However, nursing's aspirations to training based in higher education with students supernumerary to basic service provision are well known.[18] Meanwhile, the expansion of post-basic training for nurses in the higher education sector is in contrast to a reduction in social work courses in universities, and the current shift towards greater employer control over social work training.

A second but linked area of difference is in the age of recruitment. While the vast majority of qualified nurses enter training for the profession in their teens, this has always been true of only a small minority of social workers.

A third disjunction is in the sheer scale of the two occupational groups. There are in the region of half a million nurses employed by the NHS, of whom about 300,000 are qualified.[17] By contrast the number of social workers employed by local authorities is less than 100,000 even when social work assistants, home help organisers, heads of home and care staff are included, and the proportion of those employed in health service settings is very small.[15]

Fourth, in spite of a long running internal debate, social work does not share with nursing a regulatory professional council, exhibiting more ambivalence about professionalisation than its health service sister.

Finally, social work has a rather different representational structure. Both occupations have a mixture of traditional union base and a professional organisation, but the role played by the RCN within nursing is much more powerful than that of the British Association of Social Workers (BASW) in relation to social work. BASW does not share the RCN's public commitment not to strike.

Social work and nursing: a common concern with professional status

Having examined some of the central structural features of the occupations of social work and nursing, I will now turn to the detail of the argument that social work and nursing share a common problem in achieving professional status.[16] They have an apparently similar helping process, and have parallel difficulties in defining a unique knowledge base, or a precise model of health. Core values are common, though there appear to be differences in professional ethos, especially in attitudes to authority. Finally there are similar difficulties in establishing the validity of the relationship between theory and practice, against criticisms as much from within as outside the occupations. Nursing and social work also share the distinction of a defensive reaction toward doctors, jealously guarding their own status and boundaries. (See Mitchell[19] for nursing and Smith[20] for social work).

Nursing, like social work, is described as a semi-profession.[16] Both occupations have long experienced difficulties arising out of the power of doctors in medical institutions. Initially both sought solutions through the avoidance of conflict. Anne Cummins' insistence that hospital social workers 'must on no account put a foot wrong with the medical staff' (Bell[1]), sounds like an echo of Florence Nightingale's assertion that 'obedience to the doctor is absolutely essential'.[21] However, this approach is now seen as unsuccessful on various counts. As the World Health Organisation put it,

'Nursing practice and education are governed by legislation that is often archaic, determined by persons from other disciplines, detrimental to the status of the nurse and not in tune with the needs of society'.[22]

More recently a number of different strategies have emerged in nursing's struggle for status. A key component of this involves achieving increased independence from the medical profession; promoting the concept of the autonomous practitioner applying nursing theory rather than the subservient 'helpmate' triggered into conditioned response by the medical diagnosis.[14,23,24,25] However, alternative strands in the drive for status are seen in the growth of managerialism,[26] of specialisation[27] and in status by association with high technology medicine.[28] Each of these also has interesting echoes in social work.[15]

At the centre of this drive for higher professional status lies an emphasis on the nursing process and models of nursing. These are the conceptual tools to be used by the nurse practitioner, as social workers use casework or groupwork theories and models. They have a function of professionalisation in that they enable the articulation of nursing or social work activity as planned, rational, informed by theory, and capable of transmission and empirical testing.

The nursing process is a description of nursing in terms of four activities: 'assessment, planning, implementation and evaluation'.[29] Neither the process nor the language is unfamiliar to social workers; BASW's definition of social work's role in health care settings is almost identical:

'*assessing* and interpreting the patient's environment, his attitudes towards it and towards his illness, and the relationship between them, as well as *planning* and *carrying out* treatment, after-care and rehabilitation.' Quoted in Huntington,[9] my emphases.

Models of nursing are much more specific in content and vary according to the particular assumptions of the authors. The most important British model (Roper, Logan and Tierney[29]), focuses on 'activities of living' while others are described as existentialist, interactionist or systems approaches. Given the common ground between social work and nursing in respect of process, it would be instructive to explore the somewhat different approaches to generating particular models, but that is not the central purpose here.

Many of the issues faced by social work in the establishment of a knowledge base are also faced by nursing. At the heart of the matter there is the problem of the need to claim uniqueness, when nursing theory and knowledge is synthesised from a variety of other disciplines. As one author plaintively puts it,

> 'few of these in themselves are unique to nursing, yet nursing becomes unique by the unique way in which it combines these many features.' Wright,[24] and see Tibbitt[30] for social work.

For both occupations this knowledge base is predicated upon an espousal of a bio-psychosocial model of health.[29,31] However, the similarity of this concept of health may be more apparent than real. While the language of the helping process may be congruent, and while each may lay claim to a biopsychosocial and holistic model of health, the content may be more obscured than shared, more undefined than agreed.

Huntington has argued that GPs, in adopting a psycho-social as well as a bio-physical orientation to health, have focussed on inter-personal relationships rather than on relationships to the wider economic and political systems, on social psychology rather than sociology, on culture rather than social structures.[9] This is reflected too in the implicit assumptions of the Roper, Logan and Tierney model of nursing. The attention paid to the 'social' aspect of health is half that given to biology, and is essentially consensual in content, emphasising 'culture' and 'community', 'roles' and 'relationships', and paying relatively little attention to stratification and inequality.[29] Even Project 2000,[18] which has been seen as acknowledging social and material inequality, does not follow through that analysis into recommendations which impact primarily on the causes of inequality rather than service provision. (See sections 2.12 to 2.34).

This lack of precision in the 'social' analysis of Roper, Logan and Tierney's model is suggested in Savage's discussion of sexuality and nursing care. On the one hand she criticises the model for being 'very narrow'[25] while shortly afterwards she argues that 'there is a failure by nurses to use the model properly'. In concluding the discussion Savage points to the crucial issue: the ideology which is taken to underpin the model. While this remains undefined, consensus may be assumed rather than, necessarily, actual.

Huntington suggests that social workers may therefore find themselves using the same words as nurses (or GPs) but meaning different things, that the biopsychosocial model of social workers might be very different to that of other health workers. However the concept of health used by social workers is by no means agreed, and has received very little critical attention.[10,31] The literature of social work and health has been less informed by the sociological imagination than other areas of practice, and I would suggest, in contrast to Huntington, that social workers have great difficulty in applying the sociological analysis which informs social work training to their daily practice with clients. Case-based, individualistic and psychologically informed practice continues to dominate social work in spite of efforts in some quarters to find ways of thinking which link the personal and the political, private troubles with public issues.[32,33,34]

Nursing and social work theories and models also share the values of caring and coping. Caring (rather than curing) is the central nursing activity, while maximising independent coping is its central goal.[35] In the nursing process, as in social work, the client/patient is seen as an active participant rather than a passive receiver of service. This is reflected in moves away from a task based allocation of nursing time, to approaches such as primary nursing in which the patient is the oasis of allocation. Not surprisingly this has generated increased interest in the use of self in the nursing relationship,[24] and in turn calls for supervisory and case management systems more akin to social work than the traditional hierarchical approach of nursing.

If that traditional ethos is changing, it may reduce a discrepancy which appears to exist in the attitudes of social workers and nurses to authority and power, or leadership style. Nightingale and Cummins both established an ethos which avoided overt opposition to doctors. However, while nursing has a long history of emphasis on obedience within the nursing hierarchy[25] as well as to doctors, subservience has not been a feature of the socialisation into social work. As Oakley remarks,

'If Florence Nightingale had trained her lady pupils in assertiveness rather than obedience, perhaps nurses would be in a different place today'.[13]

Trevor Clay suggests that nurses are also less willing to challenge their patients than are social workers:

'Social workers are risk takers with their clients, they peel off the cotton wool and help the client and themselves face the wound and the pain. Nurses operate in a different way, less confrontational, more healing'.[17]

(Hearn makes some interesting comments about the class base of relationships within the nursing hierarchy,[16] and it would be interesting to examine the class origins of hospital social workers, to which Bell[1] makes passing reference).

Within practice and training the nursing process and nursing models have not been uncritically accepted. Again the problems of relating theory to practice sound all too familiar to a social work educator.

First, there have been difficulties over the use of language:

'terms are often obscure and incomprehensible....and words like theory, model or concept are often used confusingly or interchangeably.' Wright,[24] and see Evans[36] for a parallel in social work.

This is compounded by complaints that practising nurses have 'produced little in writing about themselves',[24] and that the development of British nursing has been dominated by ideas (and language) emanating from the United States. Thus the growing common language of nursing and social work writing - clients, change agents, models and theories of practice, assessment, planning, intervention, evaluation - may or may not reflect common thinking between practitioners, and a common task.

Second, practitioners have criticised nursing models as being unrealistic in practice and advocated only by educators who are removed from the front line of service provision.

Third, the models have been criticised as being empty, and as lacking explanatory power:

'in trying to explain everything they may explain nothing.' (Miller[37] for nursing, and see McLeod and Dominelli[33] for social work).

Sisters or rivals?

The evidence presented so far suggests that while there are significant structural and ideological differences between social work and nursing, they are less profound than the barriers to collaboration outlined by Huntington in her analysis of social work and general practice.[7] Moreover, there are signs that in a number of respects the occupations are growing closer together and that they face some similar problems. Does this therefore imply that it will be in the interests of the two occupations to form an alliance, or alliances around particular issues? Or will the increasing similarity bring growing competition or attempts at professional colonisation? There are a number of reasons for thinking that this is a possibility; centrally, that increasingly similar training and a shared community focus both have the potential for generating demarcation disputes.

For example, the training proposals in Project 2000 clearly intend to break the tradition that initial nurse training necessarily occurs in hospital, with community based training being secondary.[18] The authors rightly dispute the appropriateness of such a divide and the implication that the hospital is the main locus of health care. With the advent of the nursing process, nurses are being taught the skills of assessment, planning and intervention, they are being taught to think about the social context of the patients with whom they deal, and the communication and counselling skills to explore those issues with patients. The consequence for social workers may be that their relationships with nurses become easier. Alternatively it may be that nurses, both in and out of hospital, have greater confidence in dealing with all aspects of their patients' lives, so that the only role unique to social work becomes that of access to social services provision. At this point the residual task is little more than that of messenger. Certainly neither occupation has used the recent opportunity of rethinking its training to generate a substantial common programme; indeed there is little indication that such a possibility was ever considered.

The role of Community Liaison Sisters in hospital provides a concrete example of this point. Their task of assessing the patient and their home circumstances for community nursing services is very close to the contribution hospital social workers make in respect of social service provision. In hospitals in Dudley, the consequence is an extremely close and effective relationship between the liaison sister and the social work team, who work as powerful allies in relation to the many elements of hospital and community services with which each deals. However there can be no certainty that, as pressure on patient turnover increases, the result will be increased co-operation. It might be that the service would be better provided by a single worker able to refer to community based Health or Local Authority services. Even if not *better* provided by a single individual, it may appear to be more cost effective to hard-pressed budget holders to seek some 'rationalisation'.

Similarly the impact of the drive to close long stay hospital beds, and the press-ure towards joint planning and joint funding, may either result in closer ties, or in the 'take-over' of aspects of provision by one occupation or the other. Both the Green Paper on Primary Health Care and the Cumberlege Report on Neighbour-hood Nursing assume that social workers are not core members of the primary care team.[38,39] In a rare reference to social work, the Cumberlege Report indicated that social work and nurse assessments might be interchangeable. This might lead to bet-ter exchange but it equally might lead to one group viewing the other as redundant. Trevor Clay of the RCN explicitly points to the developing use of a

> 'more social model of care (as likely to lead to) demarcation disputes (in provid-ing services for) the mentally ill, mentally handicapped, and the long term sick and handicapped in the community'.[17]

Concluding thoughts

I have argued that the lack of attention which social work and nursing have paid to each other historically is in stark contrast to the common ground which exists be-tween them. However, it is what social work and nursing have in common as much as what separates them which is likely to result in increased conflict between the oc-cupations. Community based services, in particular, constitute 'territory' over which the occupations at the national and policy making level may well be in competition.

Paradoxically, the same forces which may generate competition between the occupations, may increase the possibility of alliances between social workers and nurses at the local level. On what basis might alliances be sought?

We now have to face an heretical question. Does it matter whether social work retains a foothold in medically dominated and historically hostile settings? In particular, if nursing adopts a concept of health and a model of the helping process which is so close to that of social work, what is social work's additional contribution to the health of patients? It is already the case that many aspects of hospital work and most primary health care settings do not have significant social work input. If nursing can be relied on to inject what Cabot described as the 'social point of view',[2] perhaps social workers would be better advised to make their contribution elsewhere. Certainly, if nursing was able to inject this perspective it would have more impact than the eighty years of social work's struggle to influence health care processes. The redeployment of hospital social workers might perhaps also do something to increase fieldworkers' awareness of the significance of ill-health in their clientele.[40]

However the definition of a 'social model of health' remains imprecise. As indicated earlier, a common language is currently being used to disguise a variety of different understandings of what makes for health. A pseudo-consensus masks the existence of practice which fails to confront factors which maintain profound inequalities in health experience and health provision. It is possible that there remains here a contribution for social work, and the necessity for linkage with elements of nursing and other interested occupations.

Finally we must return to issues of gender. From Nightingale to Oakley, those pursuing

'a definition of nursing [have found it involves] examining the relations between the role of nurse and the general position of women'13.

Carpenter argues that managerialism introduced into nursing by the Salmon Report,[26] and reinforced by subsequent developments in the organisation of the NHS,[41] was to result in the establishment of men in greatly increased numbers amongst nursing managers and leaders. Whereas there was a discontinuity between the image of a good nurse and masculinity, there is no such difficulty for men in identifying with the image of a good manager.[28] Howe draws a precise parallel for social work in discussing the disadvantaged 'career fortunes of women in welfare work'.[15]

If managerialism is one plank in nursing's drive for independence and status, specialisation is another.

'Much of the struggle of nurses for status and autonomy seems to be connected with their search for specialisation'.[27]

One route for such specialisation is through association with 'high tech' medicine, through skills in using machinery or in highly specialised procedures. While giving status, and separating out some nurses from other professionals (and from other nurses), this also moves nurses closer to the values of curative medicine - status by association with a severe sting in the tail. Both these paths to higher status seem to lead nursing away from its traditional values, values which are indelibly linked to the identification of nursing with women.[28] Hearn argues that the route to professionalisation is through the extension of patriarchy.[16]

So do nurses and social workers have an alternative? Do they either have to collaborate with medicine from a position of unequal power, embracing and reinforcing a traditional association between 'femininity' and submissiveness, or assert their independence through taking on male dominated values of managerialism or curative medicine?

Both occupations involve doing work which is low status because the values of caring and coping

'define both the identity and the activity of women in Western society'.[42,43]

As Baker Miller puts it, 'serving others is for losers, it is low level stuff'.[44]

The necessity therefore is to turn these values on their head. The possibility is to build an alliance which subsumes nurses' and social workers' *occupational* interests under their interests *as women*; which asserts the 'feminine' values of caring and coping. Such an alliance would link workers' interests in the public domain of paid work, with their interests in the private domain of family and community life. It would also operate in the material interests of women as the main paid producers of formal health care, the majority consumers of health care, and the vast majority of informal carers who bear the brunt of cuts and gaps in health care.

Such a project meets Carpenter's criterion for defending public health services as it provides the basis for action

'across the rigidly segregated occupational boundaries (while) reaching out into the community'.[28]

It also reflects Stacey's attack on male conceptions of work which split off public issues from private troubles, separate thinking from feeling, the paid work of human service workers from their personal roles within families, and givers from receivers of care.[27] Howe reached a similar conclusion in discussing strategies to combat the under-representation of women in social services management:

'The...strategy...demands that areas of work presently seen as 'female', requiring the so-called 'feminine' skills of caring, tending and domestic work receive a higher value than they do at the moment'.[15]

It also requires that what are seen as 'masculine' values are not considered a prerequisite for management.

What this would mean in practice has to be worked out at both the local and occupational level. Current debates about health and social services focus on the amounts of money spent, state versus profit making service provision, the maintenance of high technology medicine, extended forms of training and more rigorous assessment, the creation of occupational distance from new auxiliary nurses or community carers. This form of construction of the crisis in health care is likely to be damaging to women who straddle the public and private domains in quite a different way from men.[42]

Reorienting the focus of social work's collaborative effort from medicine to nursing, is then more than just a strategy for maintaining a place for social work within public health services. Alliances with nurses can involve the struggle for a redefinition of the direction of health policy, based upon the rejection of values associated with 'masculinity' and the material interests of men.

References

1. Bell, E.M. *The Story of Hospital Almoners*. Faber and Faber, London, 1961.

2. Cabot, R.C. *Social Work: Essays on the Meeting Ground of Doctor and Social Worker*. Houghton Mifflin, Tonbridge Wells, 1920.

3. Rushton, A. and Davies, P. *Social Work and Health Care*. Heinemann Educational, London, 1984.

4. Butrym, Z. and Horder, J. *Health, Doctors and Social Workers*. Routledge and Kegan Paul, London, 1983.

5. Parsloe, P. 'Foreword'. In Clare, A.W. and Corney, R.H. *Social Work and Primary Health Care*. Academic Press, London, 1982.

6. Goldie, N. 'The Division of Labour Among the Mental Health Professions - A Negotiated or an Imposed Order?'. In Stacey, M., Reid, M., Heath, C. and Dingwall, R. (eds.) *Health and the Division of Labour*. Croom Helm, London, 1977.

7. Huntington, J. *Social Work and General Medical Practice: Collaboration or Conflict*. George Allen and Unwin, London, 1981.

8. Dingwall, R. 'Problems of Teamwork in Primary Care'. In Clare, A.W. and Corney, R.H. *Social Work and Primary Health Care*. Academic Press, London, 1982.

9. Huntington, J. 'The Proper Contributions of Social Workers in Health Practice' *Social Science and Medicine*. 22, 11, 1986, 1151-1160.

10. Bywaters, P. 'Social Work and the Medical Profession - Arguments Against Unconditional Collaooration' *British Journal of Social Work*. 16, 6, 1986, 661-667.

11. Friedson, E. 'The Future of Professionalisation'. In Stacey, M., Reid, M., Heath, C. and Dingwall, R. (eds.) *Health and the Division of Labour*. Croom Helm, London, 1977.

12. Stacey, M. 'Introduction'. In Stacey, M., Reid, M., Heath, C. and Dingwall, R. (eds.) *Health and the Division of Labour*. Croom Helm, London, 1977.

13. Oakley, A. 'On the Importance of Being a Nurse'. In Oakley, A. *Telling the Truth about Jerusalem*. Blackwell, Oxford, 1986, 180.

14. Salvage, J. *The Politics of Nursing*. Heinemann, London, 1985.

15. Howe, D. 'The Segregation of Women and Their Work in the Personal Social Services' *Critical Social Policy*. Issue 15, 1986, 21-35.

16. Hearn, J. 'Patriarchy, Professionalisation and the Semi-Professions'. In Ungerson, C. (ed.) *Women and Social Policy*. Macmillan, London, 1985, 190-206.

17. Clay, T. 'The Future for Social Work and Nursing: A Royal College of Nursing View' *Social Work Today*. 18, 28, 1986, 13-14.

18. United Kingdom Central Council for Nursing Midwifery and Health Visiting. *Project 2000*. UKCC, London, 1986.

19. Mitchell, J.R.A. 'Is Nursing Any Business of Doctors? - A Simple Guide to the Nursing Process' *British Medical Journal*. 288, 1984, 216-219, and subsequent correspondence.

20. Smith, C.R. 'Social Workers in Hospitals: Misplaced Intruders or Essential Experts?' *British Medical Journal*. 277, 1973, 443-446.

21. Quoted in Kratz, C.R. (ed.) *The Nursing Process*. Ballière Tindall, London, 1979, 22.

22. World Health Organisation. *Nurses in Support of the Goal of Health for All by the Year 2000*. WHO, Geneva, 1982.

23. Dachelet, C.Z. 'Nursing's Bid for Increased Status' *Nursing Forum*. XVII, 1, 1978, 18-43.

24. Wright, S.G. *Building and Using a Model of Nursing*. Edward Arnold, London, 1986.

25. Savage, J. *Nurses, Gender and Sexuality*. Heinemann, London, 1987.

26. *Report of the Committee on Senior Nursing Staff (The Salmon Report)*. HMSO, London, 1966.

27. Stacey, M. 'The Division of Labour Revisited or Overcoming the Two Adams'. In Abrams, P., Deem, R., Finch, J. and Rock, P. *Practice and Progress in British Sociology 1950-1980*. George Allen and Unwin, London, 1981.

28. Carpenter, M. 'The New Managerialism and Professionalism in Nursing'. In Stacey, M., Reid, M., Heath, C. and Dingwall, R. (eds.) *Health and the Division of Labour*. Croom Helm, London, 1977.

29. Roper, N., Logan, W.W. and Tierney, A.J. *The Elements of Nursing*. Churchill Livingstone, Edinburgh, 1980.

30. Tibbett, J.E. *The Social Work Medicine Interface: A Review of Research*. Central Research Unit, Scottish Development Department, 1975.

31. Butrym, Z. 'Letter to the Editor' *British Journal of Social Work*. 17, 3, 1987, 305-306.

32. Evans, R. 'Unitary Models of Practice and the Social Work Team'. In Olsen, R. (ed.) *The Unitary Model*. BASW, Birmingham, 1978.

33. McLeod, E. and Dominelli, L. 'The Personal and the Apolitical'. In Bailey, R. and Lee, P. (eds.) *Theory and Practice in Social Work*. Blackwell, Oxford, 1982.

34. Bywaters, P. 'An Interactionist Approach: An Answer or Just a Better Question' *British Journal of Social Work*. 12, 1982, 303-317.

35. Henderson, V. *Basic Principles of Nursing Care*. International Council of Nurses, Geneva, 1960, 3.

36. Evans, R. 'Some Implications of an Integrated Model of Social Work for Theory and Practice' *British Journal of Social Work*. 6, 1976, 177f.

37. Miller, A. 'Theories in Nursing' *Nursing Times*. 8, 10, 1985, 14.

38. *Primary Health Care: An Agenda for Discussion*. HMSO, London, 1986.

39. *Neighbourhood Nursing: A Focus for Care* (The Cumberlege Report). HMSO, London, 1986.

40. Corney, R. 'The Health of Clients Referred to Social Workers in an Intake Team' *Social Science and Medicine*. 21, 8, 1985, 873-878.

41. *Recommendations for Action: National Health Service Management Inquiry*. DHSS, London, 1983.

42. Graham, H. 'Caring: A Labour of Love'. In Finch, J. and Groves, D. (eds.) *A Labour of Love: Women, Work and Caring*. RKP, London, 1983.

43. Graham, H. 'Coping or How Mothers Are Seen and Not Heard'. In Friedman, S. and Sarah, E. (eds.) *On the Problem of Men*. Women's Press, London, 1982.

44. Baker Miller, J. *Towards a New Psychology of Women*. Penguin, Harmondsworth, Middlesex, 1976.

Social Work in Mental Health Teams: The Local Authority Field Social Worker

Robert Brown

Introduction

This is a time of change for those local authority social workers who are actively involved in the mental health field. There is the immediate impact of the new Mental Health Acts on those who are authorised to act as Mental Health Officers or Approved Social Workers. Then there are a number of other actual or proposed changes which may significantly alter practice over the next few years: the Griffiths Report[1] and an increased emphasis on care in the community; some developments in user involvement; proposals for changes in the basic training of nurses and social workers; more referrals requesting help for elderly mentally disordered people. Together with other factors, these make for something of an identity crisis for the local authority social worker approaching the 1990s. Will the aspects of their role concerning compulsory powers dominate and get in the way of their other statutory powers and duties to provide social help and care? Or will the two areas of work develop side by side with the principle of seeking the least restrictive alternative leading to pressure for better and more varied resources? Will the social worker be one of several professionals contributing to a multi-disciplinary team, possibly co-ordinated by a doctor? Or will the role of social services care manager develop as envisaged by Griffiths?

So far as teamwork is concerned, no simple, universal model of multi-disciplinary work has emerged as yet. The social worker has to adapt to local patterns and try to find a constructive and effective way of working alongside health service employees. Other chapters in this volume examine the position of the social worker attached to a general medical practice or based in a hospital. This chapter will look at recent research and developments in so far as they affect the local authority field social worker in working as a member of any multi-disciplinary mental health team which includes doctors, nurses or other health service staff, whether it be hospital or community based. It is suggested that specialisation is already a feature of residential and day care work and that it will continue to grow in field social work for organisational reasons as well as consumer preference.

After a brief historical survey attention will be focussed on the recent mental health acts. A discussion of developments in community care will be followed by a look at the belated growth of user involvement in the delivery of services. There are significant changes in training for both social workers and nurses, some more concrete than others. The likely impact of these various issues on multi-disciplinary team work is hard to estimate and the possibilities will be considered in a final section on 'collaboration, conflict or separation?'

Recent historical background

In the five year period beginning in November 1969 there were changes in local authority and health service organisation, so that by 1975 mental health social workers found themselves employed by social services or social work departments.[2,3] Some had previously been Mental Welfare Officers, some had been hospital based psychiatric social workers, some had come from other departments, while some were emerging newly trained with the CQSW. This last group could not always understand why some of their more experienced colleagues found it so hard to identify with their employing agency, but these new 'department store' agencies were a major departure from the specialist ones which had evolved after the war. There were some attempts to pull these historical threads together in the literature, but mental health was not a high priority for local authorities in the 1970s. Patterns of service delivery tended to be dominated by other areas of work and this was reflected in the literature. Therefore, despite the earlier optimism expressed by Olsen, Mapstone, Julia and others,[3] later writers found there had been problems for mental health social workers in establishing a clear identity for themselves.[4,5] In addition, Huxley has noted recently that social workers seem to have difficulty in identifying mental health aspects of their work.[6] His contributions have been especially helpful in enabling the local authority social worker to engage in positive work in this field, especially when their initial involvement with a family has been rooted in child care legislation. Almost certainly his work, and that of Butler and Pritchard,[7] Hudson,[8] Olsen[9] and others has received a wider airing because of the Mental Health Acts of 1983 and 1984. Brandon,[10] however, has described these publications as 'the bugle call of surrender rather than that of advance' and has expressed serious concern about the impact on social work of both genericism and the new mental health acts.

The Mental Health Acts

The period which introduced the Mental Health Act 1983 and the Mental Health (Scotland) Act 1984 may prove to be a turning point in the history of mental health social work in local authorities. Bean[11] and others had identified serious problems regarding the competence of social workers carrying out duties in relation to the mental health legislation. Despite the different laws in England and Wales, Northern Ireland and Scotland the social worker has an important role in each system in, for example, assessing the need for an individual to be compulsorily admitted to hospital. Rather than reduce the social worker's role in issues of compulsion, Parliament chose to enhance it and to seek to improve competence. In the Mental Health Act 1983, covering England and Wales, section 114(2) states:

'No person shall be appointed by a local social services authority as an approved social worker unless he is approved by the authority as having appropriate competence in dealing with persons who are suffering from mental disorder.'

Section 9 of the Mental Health (Scotland) Act 1984 makes similar requirements and in many ways the two systems are closer together than before this legislation.[2] It has taken five years to set up adequate systems of training and assessment but already positive comments have been made by Louis Blom-Cooper Q.C. (who chairs the Mental Health Act Commission in England and Wales) about the competence of approved social workers in carrying out their statutory duties. He was speaking at the launch of the Law Report[12] on 11.4.1988, a document which is likely to reinforce the trend towards post-qualifying training for specialist areas of work.

A good working knowledge of the law is only a part of the training which should significantly enhance the quality of social work practice in the mental health field. Not all would share this view however and, based on his experience as a social worker in Derbyshire, Milroy[13] has argued:

'Social workers act either as welfare bureaucrats or as short term therapists competing with others to extend control over a segment of the human condition. Reductionism and multi-disciplinary work seduce us into becoming psycho-social technicians competing for control over the patient via a discrete therapy. The powers of the 1983 Act, increasing professional aggrandisement and the traditional paucity of resources, all contribute to limit "our sense of possibilities".'

The risks he identifies are real, but one could equally argue that resources going in to the new training are stimulating changes in patterns of service delivery from local authorities. Equally the quality of advice and help going to those who are detained has probably been enhanced by the new legislation. Peter Campbell[14] from Survivors Speak Out made this point as a consumer at a conference in Glasgow. This may often depend crucially on the input of hospital based social workers, either directly or through their work with nursing, medical and administrative colleagues.

As the mental health bills went through Parliament, it was far from being a foregone conclusion that health based social workers would be allowed to become approved social workers or mental health officers. There were strong arguments against this, and questions were raised about their ability to act independently of doctors in the same team. However, after some debate Parliament decided that duties connected with the use of compulsory powers should continue to be undertaken by health based social workers as well as those in area offices and elsewhere. This decision has important implications for social workers who work closely with doctors in hospitals and clinics. Firstly it acknowledges that they are not employed by the health service, which makes it easier for them to exercise independent judgement. This is not to suggest that they should be in conflict with medical colleagues, but that they have a particular role to play in the assessment of risk, social support and the need to invoke compulsory powers. Secondly it enables health based social workers to stay involved in crucial decisions regarding people they have already got to know, and therefore to provide more continuity of care. Thirdly, it makes it more likely that they will have a good knowledge of rights issues and be able to offer help in this area directly or via other staff or by putting an individual in touch with a lawyer.

In some areas hospital based social workers have taken on the bulk of the work concerning assessments for compulsory admission. Winterson[15] compared the number of applications made by hospital based social workers at the Royal South Hants Hospital in Southampton with those made by other social workers or nearest relatives. He found that of 399 applications for detention in the period 1984 to 1987:

244 (61%) had been made by hospital based social workers

112 (28%) had been made by members of the emergency duty team

33 (8%) had been made by area based social workers

6 (2%) had been made by social workers from other authorities

4 (1%) had been made by nearest relatives.

This is in an area where the acute admission wards were moved nine years ago from a Victorian hospital in the country into a district general hospital in the middle of the city. Many of the community facilities are organised from the hospital base and there are a dozen social workers situated there. Clearly, the organisation of social work services in relation to health teams and their physical location has a strong bearing on who is involved in applications. The high percentage of admissions involving emergency duty workers raises other questions about continuity of care and how these workers can maintain working links with health colleagues.

Community care

The development of community based teams in the mental health field has been somewhat patchy. Community psychiatric nurses, social workers and doctors are often still working out of hospital as in the example given above. Similarly, if it is the hospitals themselves which have moved nearer to where people live, this way of organising community care becomes more feasible. Despite the advent of a few multidisciplinary crisis intervention teams based in the community, there is little evidence yet of such services providing a real alternative to hospital admission on a wide scale, especially where the issue of compulsion has been raised.[16] However, there are various examples of local multi-disciplinary mental health services teams which have developed with local authority social workers as members.[17] It is suggested that the likelihood of these teams becoming more common will be strongly influenced by the government's response to the Griffiths Report.[1] The influence of consumer preference is less certain and will be considered in the next section.

If the number of such teams does grow there is the question of what sort of relationships will develop between the social workers and other team members. If staff currently employed by the health service are seconded to or employed by social work departments, as envisaged by Griffiths, then some of the inter-agency obstacles to team work might be removed. Whether a logical parallel development would be for hospitals to employ their own social workers is not discussed by Griffiths. The concept of the care manager organising a package of services tailored to the need of the individual might sound the death knell of the traditional multi-disciplinary team, but would it replace one form of social control with another? The Disabled Persons (Services, Consultation and Representation) Act 1986 at least gives the consumer the possibility of having a voice in service delivery.

User involvement

User involvement in mental health services is under-developed although there have been some significant examples of more consumer power in recent years. Since the World Mental Health Congress at Brighton in 1985 examples of practice in other countries such as Holland[18,19] have begun to have some influence in the United

Kingdom. Althea and David Brandon have set out some of the principles behind seeing consumers as colleagues rather than passive recipients of services determined by teams of professionals.[20] In a challenge to existing services Brandon[10] suggests that:

> 'Our services should be based on five major principles:
> - Maximising choices
> - Real integration
> - Respect for individuality, privacy
> - Participation in running the project
> - Improving relationships.'

There are now some accounts in print of the implications for local authority social workers in adopting these principles and of their impact on team work.[21,22] One particularly helpful account in this respect is that of the North Derbyshire Mental Health Services Project by Milroy and Hennelly.[23] This was originally intended to be jointly staffed and jointly funded by health and social services but in the end was sponsored solely by the social services department. One can only speculate as to whether its development according to the principles of normalisation, and its commitment to full user participation, would have been hampered or helped by joint health and social service staffing and funding.

In June 1987 the annual Association of Directors of Social Services/Policy Studies Institute seminar had as its theme 'Hearing the Voice of the Consumer' and the papers presented looked at the need for action as well as listening if social services departments were to be more responsive.[24] Issues of race and culture were among the main themes of the seminar. They have also been considered extensively by Aggrey Burke in, for example, a special journal issue on racism and mental health.[25] This volume considers how to make services more responsive to the needs of black consumers as well as the effects on teams of having members from different ethnic groups.

Consumer participation, choice and influence may be slowly developing but there is still evidence of multi-disciplinary teams acting as a block even on the basic right to obtain information about treatment plans. This problem also extends to relatives and friends. In a book aimed at these groups Kuipers and Bebbington[26] note:

> '...it may never have been made clear who within the team is responsible for saying what to whom. It may be therefore quite hard for you to get from staff any authoritative statement about what is wrong...'

Interestingly they see the social worker as a key member of the team in giving information and answering questions from relatives and friends. There is a problem here for social workers and for community psychiatric nurses. The more their work takes them into the community, the more difficult it may become for them to keep in close contact with hospital based staff and to fulfil the role of making information freely available to those in hospital or to their relatives and friends. Other ways of improving this situation include befriending schemes and advocacy schemes.[27] One way in which the consumer movement can effectively influence the way social workers operate is through their involvement in training. As an example LINK, the Glasgow based group, has contributed to basic CQSW training on the mental health sequence at Stirling University. In the practice-based part of training, involvement of users as more than passive recipients is also becoming more common.

Training

At the time of writing there is considerable uncertainty about the future of social work training. Just as the extension of nurse training to three years has introduced the prospect of new, less-qualified workers to undertake some tasks, so the proposals by CCETSW for three year courses for social workers raises questions about the appropriate level of training for social service staff working in the mental health field. Similarly, if Griffiths'[1] care managers become a reality this will have implications for training and for staffing. CSS and CQSW training are now being presented by CCETSW as equivalent. However, whatever their respective merits and faults, they are clearly different in content and this has important ramifications for mental health and the roles social workers take alongside health colleagues. Ball and others[12] identified gaps in legal training on CQSW courses, but this and welfare rights teaching is almost totally absent on CSS courses. Either a common expectation needs to be established for both courses or Mental Health Officer and Approved Social Work training will need to have a new starting point. Similarly skills in staff and money management seem to be better acquired on CSS courses and these are prerequisites for care managers.[1]

Contact with health service staff during training would appear to be a rather hit or miss affair. Brown and Pritchard[28] outlined some of the advantages of joint training but there are many obstacles to it at both qualifying and post-qualifying levels.

Where it occurs there can be significant changes in how social workers and health staff see each other,[29] but all too often a member of one group teaches the other and opportunities for learning alongside one another are missed. There are some imaginative examples of joint training in college and field but they are the exception rather than the rule.

One final influence may be that as we draw closer to Europe over the next few years there will be changes in training brought about by the need to fit into European arrangements.

These changes in training are all occurring in a short space of time. The patterns they adopt may influence the direction team work takes. Will social workers and health workers collaborate, be in conflict or go their separate ways?

Collaboration, conflict, or separation

The potential for conflict between social workers and doctors, particularly when they are involved in assessments for hospital admissions, has been well documented by Booth et al.[30] in an earlier volume of *Research Highlights*. Fisher et al.[5] concentrated their attention on area office based social workers and found:

> 'that most social workers referred to their experience of "teamwork" with other professionals in mental health as lacking or very limited. A few felt they had developed good co-operative relationships with other professionals... but the aggregate view was that, if any teamwork was desired, the social worker had to make all the running.'

They were only able to pay minimal attention to hospital based social workers in the study, but even here found considerable variation in the roles of social workers in multi-disciplinary teams.

Conflict may be associated with problems of status and leadership. Payne[31] asserts that where a team includes a doctor it:

> 'tends towards a leader-centred pattern with the doctor as leader: because others are used to a subordinate position and the group process reflects this; because doctors are either employed as independent contractors rather than employees, or are legally responsible for decisions about their patients and therefore resist the involvement of others; and also because they are usually men, and the other occupational groups around them are often women, so gender and class status backs up their dominance.'

Payne identifies strategies for improving multi-disciplinary work but is more hopeful where there is attachment rather than where contact is through a liaison scheme. Attachment or regular membership of a team would allow team building exercises, the use of outside consultants or simply occasional explanations of roles to help the team to function. If some team members did not wish to collaborate too closely they could authorise or agree to the work which was being undertaken jointly by others.

If problems of status and leadership are overcome problems may arise because of different expectations about confidentiality. The fact that team members may work for different agencies would make this even more complicated. Some of these issues are developed elsewhere in this volume and in *Research Highlights No.7*.[32]

With so much uncertainty at present concerning the future organisation of mental health services, there is also the danger that different professional groups will retrench to protect their own interests. Rather than collaborate there may be a sense of rivalry or a desire to proceed separately to carve out a clear area of work. Griffiths[1] noted the greater independence achieved by community psychiatric nurses and perhaps this is the most likely route in the immediate future. What choice the consumer will have concerning how the different professional groups work together is more open to question. In the long run how they see the different professionals' roles and how they decide to use them may be the crucial factor. In a recent survey of users' views the Falkirk District Association for Mental Health[33] found that people wanted access to doctors, nurses, psychologists, social workers, educationalists, occupational therapists and others. However, one of the main demands was for counselling services and none of the above was seen as providing this. Hawes'[34] survey of patients leaving hospital found a demand for befriending schemes, co-ordinated services, user involvement and written information.

Conclusions

The place for the local authority field worker as part of a mental health team is in a state of uncertainty. The role of the hospital based social worker changes as more people are discharged into the community and as those people who do come into hospital stay for shorter periods of time. Mental health centres and crisis intervention teams are not common. Involvement as a Mental Health Officer or Approved Social Worker requires more training and greater involvement in mental health work than hitherto, but patterns of service delivery are still settling down. Changes in training may disrupt these patterns. They may lead to more emphasis on post professional qualification work at one end and more SCOTVEC or NCVQ mental health modules at the other. The latter may fit in with demands for training by community carers just as the former have developed to meet the need for Mental Health Officers and Approved Social Workers. The government's response to Griffiths is still awaited at the time of writing.

Amidst these changes the growth in the consumer movement is timely. Peter Campbell and Ingrid Barker ran a session at the 1987 Scottish Mental Health Week Conference in Glasgow. Not surprisingly the group, who were mainly professionals, found it remarkably easy to design a system of mental health services which effectively excluded users from having any real influence.

The reverse was more difficult but the will to find ways of achieving the task was there. The Disabled Persons (Services, Consultation and Representation) Act 1986 should form part of this process. The challenge is to make it work. If it does the local authority field social worker's role in any team may become more consumer-led.

References

1. *Griffiths Report*. HMSO, London, 1988.

2. English, J., and Martin, F.M. (eds.) *Social Services in Scotland*. Scottish Academic Press, Edinburgh, 1983.

3. Olsen, M.R. (ed.) *Differential Approaches in Social Work with the Mentally Disordered*. BASW, Birmingham, 1976.

4. McGregor, C. 'Mental Health Officers and the Scottish Acts of 1960 and 1984'. In Horobin, G. (ed.) *Responding to Mental Illness*. Research Highlights, No. 11, Kogan Page, London, 1985.

5. Fisher, M., Newton, C., and Sainsbury, E. *Mental Health Social Work Observed*. Allen and Unwin, London, 1984.

6. Huxley, P. *Social Work Practice in Mental Health*. Gower, Aldershot, 1985.

7. Butler, A., and Pritchard, C. *Social Work and Mental Illness*. Macmillan, London, 1983.

8. Hudson, B. *Social Work with Psychiatric Patients*. Macmillan, London, 1982.

9. Olsen, M.R. (ed.) *Social Work and Mental Health*. Tavistock, London, 1984.

10. Brandon, D. 'The Crumbling Institutions of Mental Health' *Social Work Today*. 19, 39, 2.6.1988, 12-13.

11. Bean, P. *Compulsory Admissions to Mental Hospital*. Wiley, 1980.

12. Ball, C., Harris, R., Roberts, G. and Vernon, S. *The Law Report - Teaching and Assessment of Law in Social Work Education*. CCETSW Paper 4.1, 1988.

13. Milroy, A. 'Mutual Help Groups in Mental Health' *Social Work Today*. 19, 40, 9.6.1988, 14-15.

14. Campbell, P. 'Folk Legends from the Jungle.' Unpublished paper given at SAMH/SWSG Conference, Glasgow, 30.10.1987.

15. Winterson, M. 'Fourth Year of the Mental Health Act 1983.' Unpublished paper, RSH Hospital, Southampton, 1987.

16. Fisher, M., Barnes, M. and Bowl, R. 'Monitoring the Mental Health Act 1983: Implications for Policy and Practice' *Research, Policy and Planning*. SSRG, No.1, 1987.

17. Drucker, D. (ed.) *Creating Community Mental Health Services in Scotland*. (Two volumes). SAMH, 1987.

18. Legemaate, J. 'Patients' Rights Advocacy: the Dutch Model.' Paper delivered at World Mental Health Congress, July 1985.

19. Van Ginneken, P. 'Protecting Patients' Rights in Psychiatric Hospitals in the Netherlands'. In Jensen, K., and Pederson, B. (eds.) *Commitment and Civil Rights of the Mentally Ill.* SIND, Copenhagen, 1985.

20. Brandon, A., and Brandon, D. *Consumers as Colleagues.* MIND, London, 1987.

21. Tyson, A. 'User Involvement: Going Beyond the Buzz-Words to a New Climate' *Social Work Today.* 18, 47, 27.7.1987, 12-13.

22. Renshaw, J. 'The Challenge of Enabling the Client to be a Consumer' *Social Work Today.* 18, 47, 27.7.1977, 10-11.

23. Milroy, A. and Hennelly, R. 'The North Derbyshire Mental Health Services Project'. In Patmore, C. (ed.) *Living After Mental Illness.* Croom Helm, London, 1987.

24. Allen, I. (ed.) *Hearing the Voice of the Consumer.* Policy Studies Institute, London, 1988.

25. Burke, A.W. (ed.) 'Transcultural Psychiatry: Racism and Mental Illness' *The International Journal of Social Psychiatry.* 30, 1 and 2, 1984.

26. Kuipers, L. and Bebbington, P. *Living with Mental Illness.* Souvenir Press, London, 1987.

27. Brandon, D. 'Participation and Choice a Worthwhile Pilgrimage' *Social Work Today.* 19, 17, 21.12.1987, 8-9.

28. Brown, R. and Pritchard, C. 'Bringing Psychiatry and Social Work Together Again in Practice and Training' *Social Work Service.* DHSS, 29, 1982, 11-15.

29. Pritchard, C. and King, R. 'Changes in the Mutual Perceptions of Trainee GPs and Social Workers' *Social Work Service.* DHSS, 24, 1980, 47-52.

30. Booth, T. et al. 'Psychiatric Crises in the Community: Collaboration and the 1983 Mental Health Act'. In Horobin, G. (ed.) *Responding to Mental Illness.* Research Highlights, No. 11, Kogan Page, London, 1985.

31. Payne, M. *Working in Teams.* Macmillan, London, 1982, 105.

32. Lishman, J. (ed.) *Collaboration and Conflict: Working with Others.* Research Highlights, No.7, Aberdeen University, 1983.

33. FDAMH Internal paper in users' views of mental health centres.

34. Hawes, C. 'After-care Services for Discharged Psychiatric Patients'. In Wedge, P. (ed.) *Social Work - A Second Look at Research into Practice.* BASW, Birmingham, 1987, 59-61.

Anxiety and its Management in Health Care: Implications for Social Work

Judith Brearley

My thesis is that health settings, and hospitals in particular, are places where levels of anxiety are extremely high and have a chronic pervasive quality. It is possible to regard this state of affairs simply as an inevitable nuisance or, alternatively, to examine more rigorously the nature of the anxiety encountered, to work in the light of such understanding at various levels, and perhaps even turn a serious problem to good account.

Although there has been a great examination in writing about stress in the last few years, it is striking how little material there is relating directly to health settings. Yet as Revans observed many years ago, 'Hospitals are institutions cradled in anxiety!'[1] What follows is an attempt to explore the nature of anxiety amongst those concerned with illness or handicap and its management, patients, families and staff, to identify some of the main sources of such feelings, and then to explore both helpful and less helpful ways of coping with it.

Emphasis will be placed on those factors related to anxiety and its management which are particularly characteristic of social work in hospitals. This is not to deny that all settings share common concerns and face similar problems, but if we fail to be sufficiently specific we risk superficiality and lose an opportunity to discover the most relevant means of addressing the difficulties. The following are regarded as factors related to anxiety most likely to be encountered in hospitals, or to have certain distinguishing features there:

a) the nature and impact of the medical conditions dealt with

b) experiences of separation and loss

c) extent of uncertainty and risk, including crisis

d) institutional complexity involving particular forms of organisational structure and multidisciplinary work

e) role ambiguity (especially for hospital social workers).

All these factors interact with each other and will have differential impact, for good or ill, on patients, relatives and staff.

The nature of anxiety

One problem which should be addressed at the outset is that of terminology. This field is bedeviled by global terms in common parlance, which are rarely defined rigorously, which overlap in meaning, and whose connotations have emotional significance for most people. 'Stress' and 'burnout' are prime examples. Rather than go over this ground yet again, I propose to focus on the narrower and more neglected concept of anxiety. Anxiety can best be viewed as arising from a sense of danger. As I pointed out elsewhere,[2] the problem is not knowing who or what the enemy is, being in the realm of the unknown. Whereas for other feelings, such as depression, the trauma is in the past, it has happened, in anxiety it is felt to be in the future. The fear is that it will get out of control, and lead to panic or even total helplessness. On a more positive note, anxiety might be seen as the contemplation of an uncertainty, with the danger that something bad will happen balanced by the possibility that it will not. This opens the door for hope, and heightened motivation to work at the problem.

A characteristic of severe anxiety which has relevance for this discussion is that it gives rise to the development of defences, or, it might be said, to coping mechanisms. Denial is a common example, and like other defences it serves the purpose of giving protection against intolerable emotional pain. However, as often as not, the very defence can become a problem in its own right, causing later disturbance in functioning or relationships.

It is perhaps most usual to think of anxiety as pertaining to an individual, and not to see so clearly its presence in groups and organisations. However, this social dimension was recognised by Freud, who used the term 'affective contagion', as early as 1921.[3] Later writers, notably Isobel Menzies, have delineated the ways in which defences against anxiety can permeate institutional structure, culture and ways of working. It is significant that Menzies first conceptualised these processes through a study of stress levels in the nursing profession,[4] and later developed her ideas by means of action research in an orthopaedic hospital where young children often had to remain as in-patients for several months.[5] More recently, Obholzer,[6] in a brief paper which uses for illustration an adolescent psychiatry unit, shows how the central issues of concern in the direct work with patients can be enacted in staff conflict.

a) The impact of the medical conditions themselves

It is surprising how often the distress suffered by clients is overlooked by workers attempting to understand the nature of their own stress. Perhaps it is felt to be so obvious and inevitable as not to warrant a mention! However, I am convinced that careful attention to this factor is absolutely vital. Not only does it aid sensitivity to the predicament of those we work with, but it also helps to reduce blame and to achieve a more balanced picture of the whole situation. The implications of such a huge issue for patients, family and staff, even though interdependent, require separate consideration. Examples from the literature of each of these are offered:-

(i) Impact on patients

A social scientist and a social work practitioner, Pauline Hardiker and Vicky Tod,[7] joined forces to explore the nature of the experience of chronic illness, and the contribution of social work in such situations. They critically examine the Parsonian model of the sick role, and find that it does not seem to give adequate coverage of some important features of illness behaviour. They go on to develop a typology of illness roles, comparing acute illness, disability, terminal illness and chronic illness in terms of factors to do with the disease itself, role expectations of doctor and patient, and a range of social consequences. Chronic illness emerges as a twilight area, full of ambiguity. Conditions such as heart disease, cancer and respiratory disorders tend to be insidious in onset, fluctuating in their course, variable (even from day to day) in what is required for their management, and unpredictable in outcome. As the authors point out, 'Living with uncertainty and weariness sums up the burden of chronic illness.' Weiner's[8] description of living with rheumatoid arthritis amply and vividly confirms this. She identifies two imperatives for the arthritic, the physiological one of monitoring for pain, and the activity one of struggling to maintain a normal life, 'as two runners in a nightmare race.'

(ii) Impact on family

Rosemary and Victor Zorza,[9] in their moving account of their own daughter's terminal illness, demonstrate how out-of-phase the most caring relatives can be with the sick family member and with one another. In their case this applied particularly to crucial issues such as whether and when openly to discuss the diagnosis, decisions about treatment at home, hospital or hospice, and the varying rate at which each family member was able to come to terms with the painful acknowledgement of reality. At times both communications and relationships in the family seemed almost to reach breaking point.

(iii) Impact on staff

It is sometimes salutary to take a fairly extreme and not (to most social workers) very familiar example, as this allows the issues to be seen quite starkly; the crucial features and important insights can then be transferred to more commonplace situations. Carole Addison,[10] writing before the Falklands, Bradford and Piper Alpha, puts the spotlight on the treatment of severely burned patients, and describes in a profound way the specific stresses on social workers in Burns Units. She convincingly justifies her choice of focus on worker rather than on patient by pointing out how central is the primary need for the helper to understand his or her own reactions to suffering and the environment in which the encounter takes place, before attempting to grasp the patient's problems. She catalogues a multiplicity of difficulties including possible pre-existing individual and family problems, the circumstances of the accident, the appearance and suffering of the burned person, the possibility of death, the unpleasant treatment, and the probability of disfigurement and other long-term consequences. Words like 'catastrophic', 'tragic' and 'near-intolerable' are apt, and the worker is exposed to all this day after day. In addition there are the stresses of the environment, somewhat mitigated by group cohesion which often serves as a much-needed support system; the conflicting demands of intensive burns work with duties elsewhere, the competing priorities of technical and personal requirements of patients, the attitude of revulsion often expressed by outsiders, and the ever-present reminders of human vulnerability. The danger always exists of developing unhelpful defences against all the anxiety thus provoked, thereby becoming less useful to clients and less open as a person. More constructive ways of coping are postulated, which interestingly follow the course taken by patients and nurses who successfully adapt. These include 'emergency measures' of selective denial to conserve energy for survival followed by 'recovery mechanisms' including restoration of hope, relationships and self-esteem, leading towards partial adjustment and sometimes a sense of meaning and value.

b) Experiences of separation and loss

It is not surprising that anxiety should be so pervasive in hospital, when it is remembered that every in-patient is experiencing separation from his or her familiar environment, with all that means in terms of family, friends, routine, significant roles etc., often for a period of time which cannot be precisely defined. Compounding this problem is the fact that each patient is actually suffering a range of losses, from taken-for-granted health, through loss of mobility, function, perhaps a limb or an organ, to possible loss of life itself. At one level this is stating the obvious, but it is very common to find that health workers acknowledge such uncomfortable realities at an intellectual level only, and overlook or minimise the stark emotional implications for patients and relatives. They cannot be blamed for this, as it is impossible for any person to remain open and sensitive to intense suffering day after day without some significant forms of personal and professional support, or, alternatively but less constructively, without erecting emotional barriers against the pain.

We now know a great deal more about separation and loss than even a few years ago. Might it not be possible to use such new understanding in the service of distressed clients?

John Bowlby started studying the impact of separation on people sixty years ago. His work and that of his colleagues now conveys authoritatively the fruits of such long experience. In his most recent conceptualisation,[11] Bowlby defines 'attachment behaviour' as

> 'any form of behaviour that results in a person attaining or maintaining proximity to some other clearly identified individual who is conceived as better able to cope with the world.'

He says

> 'It is most obvious whenever the person is frightened, fatigued, or sick, and is assuaged by comforting and caregiving ... for a person to know that an attachment figure is available and responsive gives him a strong and pervasive feeling of security.'

This ethological approach stresses the survival value of such behaviour, the biological function served being that of protection. Bowlby goes on to explore its relevance for separation anxiety, showing how this is intrinsically healthy, and far from being a symptom of undue dependency.

Further debate on this theme may be found in a comprehensive examination of bereavement research by Wolfgang and Margaret Stroebe of the University of Tubingen.[12] Written from a social psychological perspective, the focus is on the death of a spouse. It makes at least two distinctive contributions to a literature which is already rich and extensive, as well as critically reviewing and comparing existing work. One concerns cultural variations in emotional reactions to loss, while the other is a detailed exploration of health consequences resulting from bereavement. An integrative view of separation and loss is taken, as evidenced in the following statement:

'By conceptualising the grief process as a form of separation anxiety, attachment theory offers a plausible theoretical interpretation of many aspects of normal and pathological grieving which have not been explained by other theories. Thus, attachment theory can explain paradoxical symptoms of grief like the urge to search for the lost person, the feeling of the presence of the deceased, or anger about having been deserted. It also allows one to identify antecedents of different forms of pathological grief. Finally it can offer an explanation for the cross-cultural invariance in the core symptoms of grief.'

A practice application of these ideas is illustrated in the work of Menzies-Lyth in the orthopaedic ward mentioned earlier.[5] Nursing staff were tending to reward those children who did not protest (an unhealthy reaction in the circumstances) and to pay little attention to the ones who were voicing their distress. The nurses gradually un-learned such responses, with the result that children were better understood and supported.

c) Extent of uncertainty and risk

Paul Brearley[13] has pointed out the significant difference between objective and subjective dimensions of uncertainty, using the phrase 'relative variation in possible loss outcomes' to distinguish risk itself from 'the feeling of uncertainty' or subjective response to being exposed to risk. In health care it is likely that these two dimensions will both be present simultaneously in large measure, as, for example, when a surgeon has to weigh the life-saving potential of an amputation against its mutilating and disabling results, while patient and family try to cope with a sense of threat and fear. In such situations, the problem is likely to be compounded by the various sorts of communication difficulties, within and across professional boundaries. The social worker, situated at the interface of medical and family systems, will have to contain his or her own anxiety in order to offer calm support to those involved.

A further potent source of risk and uncertainty is the growing incidence of violence towards social workers. Brown et al. carried out a study[14] in Wessex which identified compulsory admission of mentally disordered adults to psychiatric hospital as one major cause of violent episodes, yet few of the fieldworkers involved had been given any guidance or training in the practical management of violence. Their work usefully attempts to remedy this deficiency, by discussing not only the incidence and possible causation of violence but also ways of recognising potential violence, preventing its occurrence, and dealing sensibly with actual incidents. A number of training recommendations are made, as well as some powerful statements about the sorts of support and organisational backup which should be available.

d) Institutional complexity, involving particular forms of organisational structure and multidisciplinary teamwork

In a discussion of collaboration and conflict in relation to social work in hospital,[15] Derek Carter draws attention to differences in values, goals, role perceptions and technical procedures, and sees these as powerful potential barriers to inter-professional cooperation. He also says:

> 'The potential for conflict between the social worker and other professionals is heightened in hospitals by one of the outstanding characteristics of this particular setting, the very high level of anxiety inherent in the working situation.'

It is thus apparent that teamwork may be experienced either as a major source of necessary support, as suggested by Addison,[10] or as contributing even further to staff stress. Efforts to improve the quality of collaboration are therefore likely to help significantly, and Carter's work suggests two major ways of doing this. The first is to foster cooperation through educational ventures, aimed primarily at improving understanding of roles, and achieved by joint and mutual teaching arrangements. The second is to establish a role for hospital social work which is wider than that of caseworker and clinician. Some examples of both the problems and the potential of this approach are offered later.

The ideas of Harold Bridger[16] have relevance here. He says that as organisational complexity increases and as the environment becomes more unstable, we have to find and develop new forms of organisational membership involving 'boundary leadership', i.e. the management of both external uncertainty and internal interdependence. A greater degree of participation, flexibility, specialisation and sharing becomes necessary.

e) Role ambiguity, especially for hospital social workers

In her paper, 'The Marginalisation of Hospital Social Work - a Threat to Resist',[17] Ann Loxley reviews the changing fortunes of hospital social work since its beginnings almost 100 years ago, and the impact of successive reorganisations and professional developments since 1970. She catalogues very constructively the positive contributions of social work in health settings, but shows how these may be under very serious threat. Finally, she sounds a warning note for the whole of the social work profession unless the current trends are actively resisted. Evidence for structural marginalisation of social work in health care can be clearly seen in frozen posts, transfers to area teams, reluctance to fund services which cross territorial boundaries, and allocation of resources for statutory work with children and families as a response to public concern but at the expense of work in other sectors. Further indicators of health setting social work coming to be viewed as peripheral can be seen, she suggests, in weak support given to it by both BASW and CCETSW. The consequences must include a poorer service for vulnerable clients, a reduced opportunity for preventive work, lowered morale amongst hospital social workers, an impoverished experience for social work students facing both a shortfall and a narrowed range of placements, lessened ability to negotiate with other health professionals, and a weaker counterbalance to the social control element of social work.

Perhaps this last example is a reminder that a certain level of anxiety can be a powerful motivating force towards constructive action, by contrast with a 'head-in-the-sand' attitude which leads to passive collusion with damaging trends.

Ways forward?

For such multi-faceted and complex problems there can be no simplistic responses. A range of strategies are required at various levels which reflect the different sources and manifestations of the difficulties. Three main categories can be identified:

(i) direct individual responses

(ii) group work approaches

(iii) attempts to achieve organisational change.

These may be seen as having either preventive or remedial dimensions or both. Each will be illustrated by reference to two or three examples of current or recent work, and the strengths and weaknesses of each strategy identified.

(i) Direct individual responses to-patients, relatives or workers

Claudia Jewett's work[18] about helping children coping with separation and loss has probably been mostly used in relation to foster care, adoption and residential work, but it would be equally valuable to those working with sick and handicapped children. It is above all a practical guide, offering much advice about ways of communicating with children. Addressed equally to parents and other carers, it explains puzzling aspects of children's behaviour in straightforward language and with the aid of many examples, conveying developmental issues in a non-technical way. It enables an adult to stand in the shoes of a child struggling to come to terms with some devastating change in his life. It offers a lot of creative ideas about games and other techniques to encourage the expression and working through of deep feelings of pain, anger, ambivalence and hope.

Loss, like separation, is a field in which a vast amount of work has been done in the last 20 years, particularly in relation to bereavement. Parkes and Weiss[19] have asked whether it is possible to predict at the time of bereavement who would have greater problems of adjustment and who would cope well. It if were possible to distinguish healthy from unhealthy grieving, progress could be made in several areas. Those at greater risk could be given more help, which is an important aid to priority setting when resources are limited. There might be possibilities of prevention if we knew what circumstances gave rise to more difficulty, and helpers would be able to work in a more focussed way, with greater confidence. Of greatest interest perhaps for the theme under discussion is the work done at St. Christopher's Hospice in south London. Here, a bereavement service was introduced for those relatives identified as in need of support. A questionnaire was completed by a nurse who already knew the family, and a 'risk score' obtained by combining the responses in several key areas. Such measures, which seem at first sight fairly crude, were in fact found to have high predictive value, and have been revised to take account of increasing knowledge over the years. The extent of 'clinging and pining' proved to be the best predictor of outcome, along with the nurse's own estimate of coping ability. Systematic evaluation of the work indicated that seeking out those at highest risk and offering them counselling by trained volunteers really did improve outcome, even to the extent of reducing the incidence of suicide. The authors further suggest that understanding of these processes of recovery from bereavement might be extended to provide a model for recovery from any irremediable loss.

A thought-provoking study focussing on staff is that of Stephen Fineman.[20] He confined himself to 40 fieldworkers in five area teams but explored a wide spectrum of stress. He differentiated work-related stress from emotional demands emanating from difficulties at home, such as illness, bereavement, parenting problems or financial difficulty, and demonstrated the mutual impact of one on the other, creating in effect a vicious spiral of severely reduced tolerance of pressure in both places. Fineman used an 'intervention research' approach, aimed at working *with* his subjects through a counselling relationship while at the same time pursuing his own conceptual interests. With some social workers he moved from detailed enquiry to sharing a stress analysis summary to working out action plans and supporting attempts to implement these. Thus the chosen level of change effort was that of an individual's work realities.

(ii) Group approaches

Juanita Brown,[21] writing about the work of Play in Scottish Hospitals, describes an approach in which partnerships between parents of sick children and professionals are fostered by means of study days shared by both groups. This was not achieved overnight; indeed, the processes of enabling the sharing to take place are as instructive as their content. Substantial preparatory work was done, by means of consultations with community medicine specialists and ward sisters, and evening familiarisation sessions with parents. The latter were based on recognition that parents would not easily contemplate a frightening prospect like hospitalisation or serious illness in their child, but that, nevertheless, they would manage such a crisis better with preparation. (One in four children will have some experience of hospital by the age of seven). The focus at first was on the more familiar situation of coping with a sick child at home, play materials were used in the sessions, and information about local provision was offered. Thus parents gained understanding about how to prepare their child for a planned hospital admission, and how to support him through it and on return home by means of play. A complementary part of the process entailed study days for nursing and play staff. Gradually, the potential of bringing together the parents' knowledge of and concern for their child and the professionals' expertise in diagnosis and treatment came to be recognised, and both groups now plan the events jointly. Such sharing enables parents to utilise their resources and learn new ways of coping, and also, despite early fears, makes for more rewarding work for staff. An added bonus is that this work now provides social work students with valuable learning opportunities in the areas of communication with children, awareness of the potential of play, and resource development.

The value of these initiatives, and those of Alderson and Rees described later,[24] finds confirmation in an overview of play therapy for hospitalised children by Golden.[22] He convincingly explores the premise that

> 'play intervention for children in hospital settings is an unqualified necessity. The play therapist's puppets are every bit as important as the surgeon's knife in helping a child leave the hospital healthier than when he or she arrived.'

A very different approach[23] was used in the case of a large multi-disciplinary team which had been experiencing destructive tensions in its internal relationships. It was agreed that an external consultant should meet with the entire team at weekly intervals for a specified period, not conducting proceedings but making comment on what occurred, in such a way that the staff could see more clearly what was happening. As trust in the process developed, it was possible to discern some of the reasons for difficulty, e.g. stereotypes of prejudices firmly held by one professional grouping about another - 'doctors always make the real decisions here!' or 'Nurses are always left to pick up the pieces!' The group's own behaviour constituted very powerful evidence, to its members as well as to the consultant, of the underlying feelings. This made possible the creation of a climate of opinion in which changed and more real perceptions could hold sway. A further major anxiety for all the staff was an imminent change in senior management with attendant implications for the ethos and functioning of the unit, but this seemed to have been a taboo subject until the presence of an outsider made it safe to voice the fears directly and address the dilemmas in a mutually supportive way.

(iii) Attempts to achieve change at an organisational level

In a recent short paper,[24] Alderson and Rees look at social work practice and research in a cardio-thoracic unit in London for children with very serious conditions from an international catchment area. They identify three main social work contributions apart from practical help. These are; support to children through play therapy and to adult carers individually and in groups; gaining knowledge of the need through small-scale studies and sharing this with the hospital authorities; and finally, working for improvements in practice. They discovered that it was not sufficient to report problems and recommend improvements; they had to become change agents and go through a long process of persuading, convincing, or pressurising the decision makers about the need for change, negotiating in meetings, fund-raising and engaging in various practical tasks such as shifting furniture. The outcome was twofold. Firstly, some actual new resources were created like plans to appoint a play therapist, a redesigned admission leaflet, a display to identify staff, a story book to help prepare children and parents for heart catheterisation, and a quiet family/interview room. The second outcome, although less tangible, seemed at least equally worthwhile, and was a raising of awareness of staff about the psychological needs of child and family, coupled with emotional and practical support to meet these needs.

Cary Cherniss[25] offers a most valuable analysis of job stress and burnout, identifying contributory factors at three different levels of analysis: the individual, the work setting, and the larger culture and society. Of these, he believes that the work setting offers the most promise for effective intervention, on the grounds that it is easier to restructure a role than to change the character of either an individual or a society. In any case, he suggests, organisational design, supervision and colleague interaction are more powerful determinants of the incidence of burnout than individual personality or even perhaps than the relatively neglected area of the external environment of the agency. Programmes of staff development, including carefully thought-out systems of orientation, are seen by Cherniss as an effective and economical strategy and a good way of enabling workers to have more realistic expectations of the job. Monitoring and feedback of treatment gains can help morale, and in-service training improves staff effectiveness. An interesting recommendation is the formation of 'resource exchange networks' within and across organisational boundaries. Cherniss puts a lot of emphasis on the value of conflict resolution and organisational problem-solving, an area which in my own experience is much helped by external 'process consultation'.[21] Turning to the role structure as a major point of intervention, Cherniss advocates not only reducing role overload, ambiguity and conflict, but also finding ways to enrich the job, taking into account the individual needs and preferences of the worker. This might be done by assigning a mix of clients, balancing rewarding and unrewarding activities, allowing 'time-outs' when necessary, and building an opportunity to create new programmes into the role of every staff member. Finally the managers' needs should not be forgotten, and training, support and feedback for them should be provided.

Conclusion

There is a very strong parallel between the nature of the problems of anxiety met with in hospitals, and the processes which must be gone through to alleviate or to find constructive ways of dealing with them. The unifying factor might be seen in the principles for the management of change as articulated by Peter Marris.[26] To quote:

'First, the process of reform must always expect and even encourage conflict. Whenever people are confronted with change, they need the opportunity to react, to articulate their ambivalent feelings and work out their own sense of it. Second, the process must respect the autonomy of different kinds of experience, so that groups of people can organise without the intrusion of alien conceptions. Third, there must be time and patience, because the conflicts involve not only the accommodation of diverse interests, but the realisation of an essential continuity in the structure of meaning. Each of these principles corresponds with an aspect of grief, as a crisis of reintegration which can neither be escaped, nor resolved by anyone on behalf of another, nor hurried.'

References

1. Revans, R. *Standards for Morale*. Nuffield Provincial Hospitals Trust, 1964.

2. Brearley, J. 'Anxiety in the Organisational Context: Experiences of Consultancy' *Journal of Social Work Practice*. 1, 4, May 1985.

3. Freud, S. *Inhibitions, Symptoms and Anxieties*. Standard Edition 20, 1926.

4. Menzies, I. 'The Functioning of Social Systems as a Defence Against Anxiety' *Human Relations*. 13, 1960.

5. Menzies Lyth, I. *The Psychological Welfare of Children Making Long Stays in Hospital: An Experience in the Art of the Possible*. Occasional Papers No. 3, Tavistock Institute, 1982.

6. Obholzer, A. 'Institutional Dynamics and Resistance to Change' *Psychoanalytic Psychotherapy*. 2, 3, 1987.

7. Hardiker, P., and Tod, V. 'Social Work and Chronic Illness' *British Journal of Social Work*. 12, 1982.

8. Wiener, C. 'The Burden of Rheumatoid Arthritis: Tolerating the Uncertainty' *Social Science and Medicine*. 9, 1975.

9. Zorza, R., and V. *A Way to Die*. Deutsch, 1980.

10. Addison, C. 'Tolerating Stress in Social Work Practice: the Example of a Burns Unit' *British Journal of Social Work*. 10, 1980,

11. Bowlby, J. *A Secure Base: Clinical Applications of Attachment Theory*. Routledge, 1988.

12. Stroebe, W., and M.S. *Bereavement and Health: The Psychological and Physical Consequences of Partner Loss*. Cambridge University Press, 1987.

13. Brearley, P. *Risk and Social Work*. Routledge and Kegan Paul, 1982.

14. Brown, R., Bute, S., and Ford, P. *Social Workers at Risk*. Macmillan, 1986.

15. Carter, D. 'Social Work in Hospitals'. In Lishman, J. (ed.) *Collaboration and Conflict: Working with Others*. Research Highlights in Social Work 7. University of Aberdeen, 1983.

16. Bridger, H. *Consultative Work with Communities and Organisations: Towards a Psychodynamic Image of Man*. Malcolm Millar Lecture, Aberdeen University Press, 1981.

17. Loxley, A. 'The Marginalisation of Hospital Social Work: A Threat to Resist' *Social Work Today*. 21.1.88.

18. Jewett, C. *Helping Children Cope with Separation and Loss*. Batsford Academic, 1984.

19. Parkes, C.M., and Weiss, R. *Recovery from Bereavement*. Basic Books, 1983.

20. Fineman, S. *Social Work Stress and Intervention*. Gower, 1985.

21. Brown, J. 'Parents as Partners in the Management of Sick Children'. In De'ath, E. (ed.) *Partnership Papers*. 8, National Children's Bureau, 1986.

22. Golden, D. 'Play Therapy for Hospitalised Children'. In Schaefer, C., and O'Connor, K. (eds.) *Handbook of Play Therapy*. Wiley, 1983.

23. Personal Communication.

24. Alderson, P., and Rees, S. 'Caring for Children in Hospital: The Social Worker's Role' *Social Work Today*. 14.12.87.

25. Cherniss, C. *Staff Burnout*. Sage, 1980.

26. Marris, P. *Loss and Change*. Revised Edition. Routledge and Kegan Paul, 1986.

Change and Diversity in Hospital Social Work

John Tibbitt and Ann Connor

Writing in 1950, Jean Snelling[1] was very clear about the role of medical social work. Its purpose was

> 'to help sick people; the method is to apply the general principles of carework in the medical setting in order to assist the doctor at his task of diagnosing and treating illness ... Medical social work is an extension of the practice of medicine on the one hand and of social casework on the other.'

However she did concede that medical social work has never been static and can only be described 'as it appears at certain moments in time'. Social workers presently working in hospitals represent one of the longest established branches of the modern social work profession: the emphasis in their work now - almost 40 years after Snelling's paper - is, as we shall show, very different from the one she implies. Similarly, there can be little doubt that the role in 1950 was itself markedly different from that which had applied forty years previously as hospital almoners struggled to establish a role around the turn of the century.

Change and evolution has been and continues to be a theme running through the history of hospital social work, and has left a legacy which has contributed to the continuing debates about the scope of the social work role in hospital and the means by which it can be fulfilled. In this chapter we will be drawing on published material in order to provide a research-based perspective on some of the issues for practice and management which arise in these debates. Crousaz[2] remarked on the paucity of British research on hospital social work, a situation which has not changed substantially since. Readers will detect a reliance on recent Scottish and American research in this paper: even if the contexts in which the research has been carried out are rather different from that in other parts of the UK, we are confident that this material adequately nears on the issues to be discussed.

Historical background

First though, it will be helpful to explore a little further some features of modern hospital social work's historical inheritance in the UK, in order better to account for the potential scope that exists for the negotiation of the hospital social work role.

Almoners were first appointed in a few hospitals around the turn of the century when it became apparent that poverty was preventing many hospital patients from obtaining their prescribed treatments and thereby causing the waste of much medical effort. The almoners' essential task was to redirect those unable to support a course of hospital treatment to poor law authorities or other suitable agencies. The hospitals concerned were seeking administrative relief, although to provide it necessarily involved almoners in producing assessments of home circumstances and reporting on patients' social situations to doctors. Early almoners also took on other administrative duties. They can claim to be the forerunners of modern hospital records staff, and in the 1920s were also involved in the assessment and collection of patients' contributions to the cost of hospital maintenance through early insurance schemes.

The period between the two world wars saw the gradual recognition of the welfare role of the almoner, the demand for which was greatly stimulated during the Second World War. It was only after the war, with the development of social medicine and with it the recognition of the close relationship between social and medical factors in illness, treatment and health behaviour that the acceptance of medical social work, as it became known, as part of medical care was achieved. Its therapeutic role was increasingly recognised in psychiatry, and is now frequently 'built in' to many treatment units for physical conditions such as renal units, burns units and cancer wards.

Despite the uncertainties of the time, medical social workers were retained in the post-1948 National Health Service, and, on the reorganisation of local government in England and Wales in 1974 and in Scotland in 1975, responsibility for the service passed, with the support of the Association of British Social Workers, to the newly created local authority Departments of Social Work and their equivalents. This transfer led to the incorporation of hospital social work into service organisations which included community-based area social work teams, and social workers based in other secondary settings in prisons, schools and health centres. It added still further to the potential responsibilities of hospital social workers who could now be called upon to undertake the range of statutory functions of local authorities in child care, mental health and other welfare legislation in addition to their concern with the social aspects of health and illness of those in hospital.

Lately, as a service in, if not of, the National Health Service, it has been inevitable that the pressures on the NHS, in particular the drive for efficiency and cost-containment, should have carried implications for hospital social work. In the face of increasing pressure for hospital beds, social workers in hospitals have become, in some places at least, key people in discharge planning, and securing a co-ordinated transition from hospital to other forms of care and support based in the community.

Current patterns of provision

Within the current workload of hospital social workers there are elements from each of these stages of development. In varying degrees hospital social workers are still concerned with administrative matters to do with benefits, disabled persons' badges, or bus fares for hospital visitors; with arranging practical welfare services; with a therapeutic input to patient care; and with service planning and co-ordination. It is perhaps not surprising, in view of the broad scope for interpretation of the role on the part of social workers themselves and the other professions in the hospital setting, that there should be considerable diversity in the level and nature of social work provision to hospitals from place to place.

In Scotland approximately one in eight of all basic grade social workers and one in four of senior social workers are based in hospitals[3] - comparative figures for England and Wales are not available. They are located in some forty per cent of all Scottish hospitals,[4] although it should be remembered that cover is provided to many others on an 'on demand' basis by social workers located either in other hospital teams or in social work area teams. The issue of which base offers the most effective service to hospitals is one to which we will return.

It will be instructive first to look at the types of hospitals in which hospital social workers are located. In an earlier paper we explored the distribution of on-site social workers in Scottish hospitals.[4] Scottish hospitals are officially classified into over forty categories: these categories can themselves be grouped into those in which almost all the hospitals have hospital-based social workers, another where some but by no means all hospitals have hospital-based social workers, and a third in which none of the hospitals have on-site workers, although they may have some cover from elsewhere.

Hospitals where all or almost all had on-site social workers were predominantly larger hospitals with teaching and/or specialist units, including large teaching general hospitals, general hospitals with some teaching, large teaching hospitals for children, major teaching maternity units, and mental hospitals with major teaching units. The largest category of non-teaching hospitals in this group was non-teaching mental hospitals. It is striking that this group includes only one small category of hospitals with geriatric units, and no category of mental deficiency hospitals. Categories of hospitals where some had on-site social work staff included small and non-teaching general hospitals, hospitals with large chronic sick elements, geriatric hospitals with assessment units, long-stay mental deficiency hospitals, and non-teaching and non-GP maternity units. Those without on-site social workers were for the most part GP cottage hospitals of various sorts, convalescent units, and a small number of specialist hospitals. Many hospitals in those categories were small, most having less than one hundred beds and many only between thirty and fifty.

We were also able to look at the level of social work provision to these hospitals as measured as a ratio of hospital social workers to the number of occupied beds (not an ideal indicator, but alternatives are hampered by lack of data), and at the seniority of the social work staff available. For these categories of hospitals where at least some have on-site social work staff, the findings are summarised in Figure 1. The picture presented highlights the wide diversity in the distribution of hospital social work staff, not only between categories of hospitals but within any particular category too.

It appears that there has been some detectable shift in the distribution of hospital-based social workers in the period for which local authorities have been responsible for the service, away from large general teaching hospitals, large teaching hospitals for children and mental hospitals towards mixed specialist hospitals, long-stay geriatric hospitals, non-teaching and non-GP maternity hospitals and mental deficiency hospitals. But it was the case that by 1982, whilst most categories of hospital with social workers had gained in absolute numbers, the categories of hospitals which local authorities inherited which were well-endowed with hospital social workers continued to attract a disproportionate number of new posts. Overall, our analysis concluded that distribution of hospital social work remains heavily linked with historical inheritance, which in turn had associated posts disproportionately by patient group, status of the hospital, and hospital size.

This diversity is probably the inevitable outcome of the process of allocation of new posts undertaken by local authority managers. In the absence of generally accepted criteria for the allocation of hospital social work resources, allocation decisions have been shown to be the result of a pragmatic weighing of a number of factors concerned with the staffing and organisation of the hospital, the position in the social work department, and the prevailing beliefs locally of the role of hospital social work.[4] A more systematic approach to the deployment of hospital social work resources, essential if the effectiveness of their input is to be maximised, requires careful scrutiny of the impact of hospital social work in different settings, and of the

Distribution of Social Workers and Hospital Classification

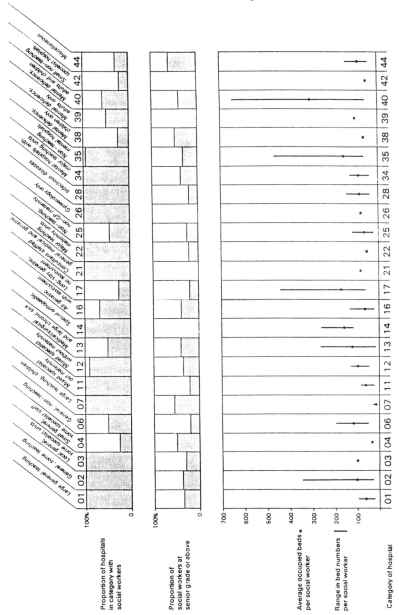

workload these settings may be expected to generate. The rest of this paper will be concerned with research material relevant to these issues.

The content and effectiveness of hospital social work

If change and diversity are the outstanding features of hospital social work in the UK, what do we know about the content of the work undertaken by hospital social workers and its particular contribution to the well-being of patients and their families? There are two principal sources of research material to draw upon, namely time-use studies and evaluations of practice in specific hospital settings.

Time-use studies

There are very few published time-use studies in Britain. Since Butrym's study 'Medical Social Work in Action'[5] published in 1968, we are aware only of studies in Manchester[6] and in Scotland,[3] and because of differences in the way material was analysed it is not easy to draw comparisons between them. It is understood that a few other Social Service Departments have reviewed their work in similar ways for internal planning purposes, but the findings have not been given a wider airing.

The Manchester study surveyed the activities of almost all hospital social workers in the area (99 of 101) who were spread across a wide range of medical and psychiatric settings. The study shows clearly that differences in patterns of work existed between different units and specialisms, both in the use of time by hospital social workers and in the types of help given to clients. Medical units, for example, gave short term intensive help characterised by an emphasis on emotional and therapeutic help, whilst in Psychiatry Units work was long term with a high proportion of cases, and psychiatric social workers undertook the greatest amount of direct work with relationship problems, concerning both mental/sexual and parent/child relationships. In our study in Scotland, which was confined to paediatric and geriatric settings, whilst the range of tasks undertaken by social workers in the two medical settings was very similar, there were some differences in the balance of time spent on specific aspects. In geriatrics, for example, relatively more time was spent in direct work with clients, whilst in paediatrics relatively more was spent in formal meetings such as case conferences. The range of issues addressed by the social workers also varied within a common range, again reflecting the different needs of their clients, which are in part determined by the patients' personal characteristics - such as age or lifestyle - and the nature of their illnesses.

There is also research evidence about the effects of higher social work staffing levels in hospital units. An increased level of social work cover is associated with an improved quality of service to clients. Social workers in the higher staffed teams in the Scottish study were able to spend more time in direct work with clients and other case-related work; were more often able to work to a planned care strategy; more often provided a liaison role for other hospital or community-based social workers, and had a greater opportunity to use specialist social work skills in their work. This improved service did not only result in benefits to the clients, however. Other professionals within the hospital and working in the community - including other social workers - had better information and could plan their work with these patients more appropriately. Also the more extensive social work input, especially to discharge planning with elderly clients, was associated with overall resource savings through earlier discharges and reduced likelihood of patients returning to the hospital when arrangements for community based support proved to be insufficient.

Practice in specific settings

Much of the most relevant writing on this topic has been in the United States, where open debate within the profession about the remit of hospital social work is better established, and there is a longer established tradition of practitioner-research. As a consequence there is a considerable volume of American literature both describing and systematically evaluating the consequences and impact of the social work input to health care. Two journals both launched in the mid-1970s are devoted to health care and social work, and over the past five years almost half the articles published have been reporting research findings, introducing research-based planning and evaluation tools for practitioners or providing an overview of recent research work on a specific area. Some seventy per cent of these studies have had a strong practitioner input while the remaining thirty per cent have been carried out by external agencies such as universities, or federal or state government departments. Typically, the practitioner studies are based in a single hospital or unit, often focussing on the characteristics or views of clients or aspects of social work intervention in a particular medical specialty. There is a widespread balance between mental and physical health care, and the physical medicine specialisms cover a wide range, for example oncology,[7,8] gynaecology and obstetrics,[9] paediatrics,[10] and cardiac[11] and renal units.[12] As might be expected, some studies are based on small samples or are very specific to that setting, but the great majority have been structured and carried out in a rigorous way that gives a wider relevance.

In contrast, in Britain there has been no specialised publication focusing on this range of professional issues since the Journal of the Institute of Medical Social Work (formerly the Institute of Almoners) ceased publication in the late 1960s. Since then hospital social work has had to compete with other aspects of social work in the British Journals. The emphasis in British studies is firmly on mental health care, reflecting the more established body of psychiatric social work practice, and when the studies focusing on community-based rather than hospital-based care are set to one side the number of studies evaluating the social work contribution to in- and outpatient care of ill and disabled people is very small indeed. Relative to population rather more work appears to have been done by researchers and social workers in Northern Ireland, perhaps reflecting the different organisational structure of health care and social services in the province.[13]

The reasons for this larger body of American work are well recognised - the different way in which health care is funded in the United States; the direct employment of social workers by hospitals and non-profit making organisations, and the need for the social workers to justify their work to their employers and non-social work colleagues; the postgraduate training of social workers which involves carrying out original research; and the way in which this is enhanced by close links between hospitals and university medical and social work schools where, for example, medical colleagues will also be carrying out and publishing research work. Throughout the American literature, the researchers comment on the need to demonstrate the work of the social work department to colleagues within the hospital, and to promote the value of the social work contribution for both clients and the host agency. Specific studies identify the areas of work where the social work contribution has been more or less well received and the factors behind the attitudes of other professionals, and have used this to suggest ways of promoting the social work contribution.

One study of patients who had experienced serious heart attacks which looked at the support available from their informal networks and from health care and other professionals, and at their unmet needs, found that hospital social workers were the only, or best placed, people to enhance the support given by the patient's informal network (which was the main or sole source of support for most people); to help the patient deal with the emotional impact of the crisis, especially in the medium - longer term; to provide help in particular areas not addressed by friends and relatives such as tackling the financial consequences of the person's medical condition; and to help the family tackle the issue of their long-term adjustment to the patient's subsequent ill-health. This study also identified ways in which the social workers could reach patients currently slipping through the referral system and extend the range of support offered to meet patients' needs.[14] All these points closely reflect the findings of our own study of the work done by hospital social workers in Scotland, even though this study looked at quite different medical settings.

The social work input has also been seen to assist the medical care given to patients. Thus in a study of social work intervention with families of children suffering from leukaemia, as well as providing emotional support to families when dealing with the shock of the diagnosis and in some cases, later, with the child's death, and also with the wider implications of the situation for other aspects of family dynamics, the social work input helped the children and parents co-operate with the medical care. Specifically, the families with whom the social worker was involved had easier, more equal relationships with the medical and nursing staff and were more likely to maintain regular attendance at out-patient clinics over several years.[15] Similarly, social workers caring for renal patients have demonstrated to nursing and medical staff that families with poor relationships are less likely to cope with long-term home dialysis - to the extent of some patients dying unnecessarily - and have helped health care staff overcome their reluctance to initiate or suggest 'interference' in this area.[12,16]

The complexity of the interaction of illness and family dynamics is also well illustrated in the study by McAuley et al. of the social work task at an acute psychiatric hospital in Northern Ireland. Here, it found that the most prevalent social work problem at the time of clients' admission was in their family relationships (fifty-five per cent of all people admitted over a six month period), while the next most frequent problem was that of loneliness and social isolation.[13] The interaction of factors associated with health and pre-existing social work problems was also found to be shared by many of the families with children and elderly people in the general medicine settings featured in the recent Scottish study.[3] However McAuley and her team also highlighted the similarities in the ways they went about dealing with their clients' problems and the social work task undertaken in area teams, despite the rather different characteristics and needs of the clients concerned, resulting in a different context and focus in the shared tasks such as mobilising practical services, offering information and advice and undertaking assessments.

Work related to patient discharge has always been a key aspect of the professional role in both the United Kingdom and United States of America, and increasing financial pressures have made this one of the major issues of concern among hospital social workers in America.[17] However, other more positive aspects of discharge planning have been described, especially for groups of clients whose wish to return to the community is strong, such as severely disabled and frail elderly people. By emphasising the client's social needs rather than his medical functioning, social workers can to some extent shift the focus from the hospital's perspective (clearing beds) to the client's perspective (reassessing his lifestyle, adjusting to loss and planning for the future). Here the contribution of social workers has been to enhance clients' control over the timing and circumstances of their discharge to the community and to help families build on their previous relationships to take on new roles imposed by the consequences of illness or injury.[18] Indeed, much of the American research work related to this area of client care is concerned with evaluating ways of predicting at an early stage which patients are likely to experience problems at the time of discharge. The wider impact of the social work contribution in making other service providers more aware of clients' needs after discharge from hospital has also been noted. In this, staff may be seen as working within and developing the traditional advocacy role of hospital social workers.[19] In all these instances of work in discharge planning the work described in the American studies has many similarities with the work of staff working with elderly clients we have described elsewhere.[3]

Cost containment

Despite the fundamentally different methods by which health services are funded in the USA and in Britain, they share a number of common problems, one of which relates to the need to curb escalating costs arising from advancing medical technology and rising demand in the light of demographic change and increasing expectations in the population. Whether as a result of pressure from the private health insurance industry or of Government policies to constrain public expenditure, health service agencies have had to scrutinise their practice to justify the service input in the response to the introduction of target periods of medical care for particular diagnostic categories of illness, and to improve the efficiency with which expensive resources are used. It is in part due to such pressures that there are clear trends to shorter in-patient stays, greater patient turnover, and rapidly increasing use of day and out-patient treatment wherever possible.

Hospital social workers, particularly in the US where social services departments in hospitals, unlike their counterparts in the UK, are on the hospital payroll, have inevitably been caught up in these scrutinies, and in their turn been required to demonstrate the cost-effectiveness of the social work contribution both to patient care and to overall hospital performance. The response can be seen in two main areas: first, the increasing adoption by hospital social work teams of techniques for quality assurance, and second, with studies of the hospital social work contribution to minimising lengths of stay in hospital mainly, although not exclusively, by speeding up hospital discharge. For a good review of the first of these see Coulton:[20,21] here we will concentrate on the second.

Delayed discharge and 'bed blocking' are familiar problems in hospital settings. A 'bed blocker' is someone who has been in hospital for a period of time, who, in the opinion of the medical and nursing staff, no longer requires the facilities provided by the hospital, and who cannot be discharged because there are no adequate arrangements for continuing care elsewhere. The majority of blocked beds are occupied by elderly people.[22] Studies have identified a number of factors which contribute to improving the prospects of early discharge for elderly patients. Consistently, these studies point to the importance of early multi-disciplinary assessment, early planning of discharge arrangements, and an early social report.[23] They emphasise the need for good communication between members of the multi-disciplinary team and the patients' families,[24] and recognise that the social needs of patients should receive as much attention as their medical problems.

Hospital social workers, as we have seen, are key actors in all of the processes associated with securing the earliest appropriate discharge of hospital patients. In a controlled experiment, Boone et al.[25] have demonstrated the impact of early social work intervention on length of stay of patients on orthopaedic wards. They showed that for all diagnostic categories, patients in the experiment group spent, on average, fewer days in hospital than did patients in the control group.

When costs were attached to the days 'saved', the study was able to demonstrate the cost-effectiveness of employing social work staff on the ward. Our own study showed that, within the Scottish Health Service category of geriatric hospitals from which our sample was selected, the presence of significant hospital-based social work was consistently associated with hospitals with the shorter average lengths of patient stay.[3] Hospital social workers, whilst they cannot claim the sole credit for reducing hospital stays and hence containing health service costs, demonstrably make a real contribution in cost-effectiveness terms to this process.

Two caveats should perhaps be entered here. First, there are suggestions that some social workers feel uncomfortable in the role of 'bed clearance assistants',[26] and are reluctant to operate a placement service for private nursing and residential homes. On the other hand, Blazyk and Canavan[27] have recognised the therapeutic possibilities inherent in the task of discharge planning, seeing it as an opportunity to help clients and their families through the changes in social role definition which may be required as a result of illness or disability.

Second, questions have been raised about the necessity of after-care placement requiring the skills of a trained social worker. Some health authorities are experimenting with the provision of their own placement services in a bid to reduce costs even further. Comparison of the quality of service received under these different modes of service provision have yet to be made.

Increasingly, the wider concern with cost effectiveness of the social work service itself has been gaining prominence, and this issue has been tackled by the research studies. Thus a study was conducted in one State of the changes in the departmental structure and role of hospital social workers over a six year period in the late 70s and early 80s when greater cost control was being introduced, causing concern that the social work contribution might be restricted or reduced. It was found that although there had been a reduced service in some specific areas especially services to discharged patients:

> 'the departments have by and large sustained or enhanced their position with regard to the professionalisation of the department, staff size, involvement in patient care, and participation in hospital decision-making'.[28]

Similarly, an evaluation of a structured management approach intended to introduce greater accountability into the work of a large hospital's social work department highlights both the perceived need to carry out and publish work of this type. Here, it was found that as well as helping social workers to devote more time to patient care and monitor the effectiveness of their work with specific clients, the management system had validated professional social service standards to the hospital administration, led to improvements in the clinical and administrative autonomy of social workers, enhanced the overall patient-care decision making within the hospital, and benefited the social work department and other parts of the hospital by providing a mechanism for handling management and organisational conflicts which had previously taken up an undue amount of time. Here again, in a situation where cost-effectiveness was becoming a crucial factor and services cut back, the social work department was not reduced but instead was able to expand.[29]

Social workers have become involved in developing appropriate means of costing and evaluation of the social work contribution to patient care and other aspects of the hospital's functioning, recognising that if the profession does not undertake this task other professions, using different criteria and assumptions, will impose other costing mechanisms upon them.[30]

There are also accounts of how social workers have used the findings of their own and other researchers' studies in the smaller scale context of particular specialisms, again to develop ways of planning and delivering their social work services more effectively. Examples have included identifying clients who have most need of a social work service, the most appropriate form of input for families in different circumstances, defining social work goals for intervention and avoiding or minimising unproductive interventions. Here also, social workers have found that in adopting a more structured approach this has in turn led to improved inter-disciplinary working with medical and other professional staff and to their social work team receiving more appropriate and better presented referrals.[31,3]

Allocating hospital social work staff

We described earlier the very diverse pattern of hospital social work staffing which characterises the service both in the UK and in the USA. In Britain there is no official guidance on the determination of staffing levels in hospital settings. Recently, though, there have been attempts to derive predictive models both to calculate required staffing levels in particular hospital settings and/or to achieve equity in the distribution of available resources between settings.

Krell and Rosenberg, following a period of research in American hospitals, have produced what they refer to as a 'usable guide for staffing in-patient service areas of acute hospitals'.[32] Their basic assumption is that required social work staffing will be a function of the size of the hospital patient population, the need in the patient population, and the extent of the social work services to be offered in the setting. Their formula is as follows:

$$\text{Staff needed} = \frac{\text{No. of beds} \times \% \text{ of patients requiring SW}}{\text{Staff caseload ratio by functions carried out}}$$

To support this formula they provide a list of nineteen potential social work functions for hospital workers and from their research derived three staff caseload ratios (1:35 cases, 1:25 cases, 1:15 cases) depending on the number of social work functions undertaken. Equity between different settings can also be achieved if actual staffing in each setting stands in some fixed ratio to the social work staffing figure predicted on the basis of the model. Flowers[33] has described an approach in an English authority which has some similar features to the model described.

Christ[34] in the US and Law and Huxley[35] in Britain have both demonstrated a strong correlation between patient turnover and the amount of direct social work time per patient. Law and Huxley used regression analysis with health and social work workload data to account for the variation in staffing levels. It showed that throughput was the most important variable in the 'explanation' of staffing variation. When variables closely related to throughput were used in the regression equation a three variable equation was produced which accounted for 'almost all' variation in staffing levels. Their model is of the form:

Staff level = a + b₁ (case contact time) + b₂ (no. of cases seen per year)
where a, b_1 and b_2 are derived from the regression equation in the light
of parameters drawn from local data.

The extent to which such models as these can provide universal predictors of staffing needs requires further research; such work deserves some priority if managers are to be confident of allocating resources at their disposal to the best effect.

Organisation of the social work service

Given that resources are likely to be under pressure and scrutiny, the need to find the most appropriate way of organising these services to ensure the greatest impact becomes particularly important.

There are two aspects of the organisation of social work to hospitals which are of concern here. First is the issue of whether the service should best be provided by on or off-site social workers, and second is the question of how to secure the most effective working links with medical and nursing services within the hospital. In important ways, these two issues are linked: both are concerned with serving the most effective organisational arrangements which will maximise the effectiveness of social work input for clients and also the efficiency of inter-agency working between hospitals and community-based services.

For most patients, a period of hospitalisation represents a phase in a treatment career which is likely to end with discharge back to the community, either to his own home or to a substitute home, if the nature of the illness has been such as to alter permanently the practicality of living in the previous home environment. It is important from the patient's point of view that these transitions into and out of hospital are managed in a co-ordinated way, that choices are explored in order to determine the most appropriate forms of support, and that continuity of care from one phase to the next is maintained. From the services' point of view it is important to secure the efficient movement of the patient between services at the time appropriate to patient need so as to ensure that only the maximum input necessary to meet patient need is provided and unnecessary use of expensive resources is avoided.

The key issues are therefore that the service should be organised in a way that provides:

- easy access by potential clients, and/or their participation in decision-making about their future care as far as possible;
- good on-going liaison between the hospital and community services; and
- good liaison between the social work and health care services.

In our recent research which examined the service given by hospital based social work teams with different levels of staffing and by area teams on an 'on request' basis, the social care given to patients by social workers and other professionals was notably better when it was based at the hospital. In particular, when the potential clients were reliant on staff from an area team:

- fewer people who appeared to need a social worker's input received it;
- patients and their families had less opportunity to plan their own future;
- ward staff and community based professionals had little information about the care which the others had been or would be providing;
- there were frequent delays in cases which were referred being picked up for assessments for services; and
- people were less likely to receive community services on discharge and those which were delivered were again prone to delays, thus leaving the person inadequately supported for that initial, vulnerable few days.[3]

The reasons for this are complex, involving such factors as the relative priorities of competing demands within the area teams' caseloads, the low risk of people remaining in hospital coming to any immediate harm when compared to their counterparts already at home, perceptions on the part of social workers and health care staff about the other's roles and organisational tensions between the services, and the physical distance between the area office and hospital. However the practical consequence was that the interests of the hospital patients - including those who were already social work clients - were not fully met. Indeed such people were better served and their community-based social worker's job was eased when there was a hospital social worker who could provide a channel of communication with the medical services and help the other social worker to co-ordinate the hospital and community services around the client.

However the study also highlighted ways in which the social work service within a hospital team could be more or less effectively organised. As has been noted above, the service improved when the level of staffing increased. Even within this pattern, however, there were marked improvements when specific social workers worked with the consultants and other staff on each ward or unit as part of an interdisciplinary team, in contrast to the model where the social work service to the hospital was dealt with by the social work team on an intake basis. In the former situation the type of advantages gained by the social workers based on site were again noted. In particular the social workers could undertake more independent case finding and were less reliant on other staff's perceptions of their role; they took on a wider range of cases and could use specialised social work skills to greater effect; and other staff had a better understanding and appreciation of the social work role because they had experience of the consequences of this intervention through regular feedback.

Most of these advantages stemmed from regular planned, structured contacts such as participation in ward social rounds, which complemented the frequent informal contacts which stemmed from the physical proximity of the people concerned. It may well be that this method of working could be adapted and incorporated into those situations where it is decided that the social work service should be provided by an area team, for example at the smaller hospitals in rural areas mentioned earlier in this paper.

Conclusion

This paper has commented on some of the key features of the contribution made by the social work service to health care in hospitals and the implications of the way in which this is organised. We believe that these are crucial to an understanding of the stage to which this part of the social work profession has developed so far, and to any consideration of the direction it is likely to take in the future.

The hospital social work service has demonstrated its value in meeting the social care needs of people who need hospital care because of their illness or disability and in supporting the wider family network through what is often a period of great stress. It has been seen to complement and enhance both other social work inputs and the health care provided for its clients. Lastly, the service has been seen to justify itself in resource terms, both by helping to ensure the most efficient and effective use of other services and in terms of its own cost-effectiveness.

However, despite this, hospital social workers in many parts of Britain and elsewhere feel themselves to be under pressure, and to be misunderstood both by their departmental colleagues and managers and by the health care staff with whom they have to work.[36] It may be that if the hospital social work service is to survive and develop over the next forty years more work needs to be done by social workers themselves to assess the work which they do and its outcomes, to consider how to refine and improve that input still further, and then to disseminate these findings to inform the debate about what type of service should be provided to people when they need hospital care.

References

1. Snelling, J. 'Medical Social Work'. In Morris, C. (ed.) *Social Casework in Great Britain*. Faber and Faber, London, 1950.

2. Crousaz, D. *Social Work: A Research Review*. HMSO, London, 1981.

3. Connor, A., and Tibbitt, J. *Social Workers and Health Care in Hospitals*. HMSO, Edinburgh, 1988.

4. Tibbitt, J., Ulas, M., and Connor, A. *Features of the Deployment of Social Workers in Scottish Hospitals in 1982*. Scottish Office Central Research Unit, 1982.

5. Butryim, Z. *Medical Social Work in Action*. Bell, London, 1968.

6. Manchester Social Services Department. *Hospital Social Workers: A Study of Patterns of Work and Use of Time*. SSD, Manchester, 1981.

7. Staley, J. et al. 'Cancer Patients and their Co-workers: a Study' *Social Work and Health Care*. 13, 1, 1987.

8. Davidson, K. 'Social Work with Cancer Patients: Stresses and Coping Patterns' *Social Work and Health Care*. 10, 4, 1985.

9. Kohn, I. 'Counselling Women who Request Sterilisation: Psychodynamic Issues and Interventions' *Social Work in Health Care*. 11, 2, 1986.

10. Waldron, J., and Assayama, V. 'Stress, Adaptation and Coping in a Maternal-Fetal Intensive Care Unit' *Social Work in Health Care*. 10, 3, 1985.

11. Dhooper, S. 'Family Coping with the Crisis of Heart Attack' *Social Work in Health Care*. 9, 1, 1983.

12. Peterson, K. 'Renal Units: Psycho Social Adjustment of the Family Caregiver: Home Hemodialysis as an Example' *Social Work in Health Care*. 10, 3, 1985.

13. See for example McAuley, P. et al.: 'The Social Work Task in an Acute Psychiatric In-Patient Unit' *British Journal of Social Work*. 13, 1983, and the Social Work Advisory Group series published by DHSS.

14. Dhooper, S. 'Social Networks and Support during the Crisis of Heart Attack' *Health and Social Work*. 9, 4, 1984.

15. Kupst, M. et al. 'Strategies of Intervention with Families of Paediatric Leukemia Patients' *Social Work in Health Care*. 8, 2, 1982.

16. Palmer, S. et al. 'Helping Families Respond Effectively to Chronic Illness: Home Dialysis as a Case Example' *Social Work in Health Care*. 8, 1, 1982.

17. See for example the New Focus Interview in *Community Care*, 26 May 1988, p.7.

18. Blazyk, S., and Canavan, N. 'Managing the Discharge Crisis Following Catastrophic Illness or Injury' *Social Work in Health Care*. 11, 4, 1986.

19. Lurie, A. 'The Social Work Advocacy Role in Discharge Planning' *Social Work in Health Care*. 8, 2, 1982.

20. Coulton, C.J. *Social Work Quality Assurance Programmes: A Comparative Analysis*. National Association of Social Work, Washington DC, 1979.

21. Coulton, C.J. 'Quality Assurance for Social Services Programmes: Lessons from Health Care' *Social Work*. 27, 5, 1982.

22. Ham, R. 'Speeding up Discharge' *The Health Service Journal*. 14 April, 1988.

23. Burley, L.E., Currie, G.T., Smith, R.G., and Williamson, J. 'Contribution from Geriatric Medicine within Acute Medical Wards' *British Medical Journal*. 279, 1979.

24. Murphy, F.W. 'Blocked Beds' *British Medical Journal*. 274, 1977.

25. Boone, C.R., Coulton, C.J., and Kello, S.M. 'The Impact of Early and Comprehensive Social Work Services on Length of Stay' *Social Work in Health Care*. 70, 1, 1981.

26. Westland, P. 'Social Work in a Quandary' *Health Service Journal*. 26 May, 1988.

27. Blazyk, S., and Canavan, M. 'Therapeutic Aspects of Discharge Planning' *Social Work*. 1985.

28. Schlesinger, E., and Wolock, I. 'Hospital Social Work Roles and Decision-Making' *Social Work in Health Care*. 8, 1, 1982.

29. Spano, R., and Lund, S. 'Productivity and Performance: Keys to Survival for a Hospital-based Social Work Department' *Social Work in Health Care*. 11, 3, 1986.

30. Haber-Scharf, M. 'Costing Social Work Services in a Hospital Setting' *Social Work in Health Care*. 11, 1, 1985.

31. Sulman, J., and Verhaeghe, G. 'Myocardial Infarction Patients in the Acute Care Hospital: A Conceptual Framework for Social Work Intervention' *Social Work in Health Care*. 11, 1, 1985.

32. Krell, G.I., and Rosenberg, G. 'Predicting Patterns of Social Work Staffing in Hospital Settings' *Social Work in Health Care*. 9, 2, 1983.

33. Flowers, J. 'Can we Develop an Allocation Formula for Hospital Social Work?' *Social Work Service*. 1981.

34. Christ, W.J. 'A Method of Setting Social Work Staffing Standards within a Psychiatric Hospital' *Social Work in Health Care*. 8, 2, 1982.

35. Law, E., and Huxley, P. 'Models with National Potential' *Health Service Journal*. 27 November 1986.

36. See for example the recent moves by Southwark and other Social Services Departments to greatly reduce the level of social work cover to hospitals, especially those treating a high proportion of patients from outwith the local area.

Health Assessment of the Elderly: A Multidisciplinary Perspective

Phyllis Runciman

The provision of appropriate health care for the growing number of elderly in Britain is presenting interesting challenges and questions for the latter part of the twentieth century.

On the one hand, myths of ageing need to be challenged vigorously;[1] many old people continue to lead enjoyable and stimulating lives and are making a major contribution to society, to communities and within families. On the other hand, there are many who are undoubtedly at risk and who face actual and potential threats to health from a variety of sources - physical, emotional, social and environmental. Assessment of old people at home, to identify both strengths and threats to health, is therefore an area of shared and growing concern to those who work in health and social services and in the voluntary sector.[2,3,4,5]

The topic 'health assessment' is complex and prompts many questions. What is meant by the term 'health'? What should be assessed? Which old people should be assessed, how are they to be identified and by whom? How should an assessment be carried out? How do health and social service workers feel about assessing old people? And how do old people themselves and their carers feel about assessment and its value?

A number of these questions were addressed in a collaborative project carried out by a general practitioner-health visitor team.[6]

Study aims

The research study had two aims:

1. To describe the scope and content of health assessment of older people at home as perceived by different professional groups and by older people themselves.

2. To describe the views and feelings of different professional groups towards visiting and assessing the health of older people at home.

The original intention had been to devise and test a standard 'package' for assessing old people. This was not done for two reasons. First, it seemed that there might be considerable resistance in teams and from individuals to the use of such packages. Comprehensive and standardised proforma, which are generally long and complex, can be of use for large scale identification of need; they are less useful and less appropriate for sustained health care provision by teams and by individuals. Second, it was felt that the ambivalence which has long been apparent amongst professionals about work with old people merited further study.[7,8,9]

TABLE 1
Study sample

Category	Number
Health visitor students	43
Experienced health visitors:	
Fieldwork teachers	33
Others	20
District nurse students	24
Experienced district nurses	19
General practitioner trainees	50
Experienced general practitioners	26
Physiotherapy students	20
Occupational therapy students	9
Social work students	9
Home care (home help) organisers	34
Elderly people	31
TOTAL	318

Sample

As so many groups are involved in assessing the elderly at home, the aim was to include a cross-section of student and experienced care workers and a number of elderly people (Table 1). All were drawn from the East of Scotland.

The total sample was large; $n = 318$. Claims cannot be made, however, about the representativeness of these groups. The experienced health visitors, district nurses and general practitioners were self-selected as being interested in the care of the elderly. The occupational therapy and social work student groups were small and self-selected from larger class groups. The old people were attending two day centres; but as 'old people' are a heterogeneous group, it is not known whether they were in any way representative of old people in general. However, the health visitor, district nurse and physiotherapy student groups represented total class groups; and the fieldwork teachers, trainee general practitioners and home care organisers were the majority for the geographical area; these groups may therefore be more representative of the total populations. Biographical questionnaires indicated that there were major differences between and within study groups in educational and professional background and in work experience. Some had had considerably more opportunity than others because of age and life experience to learn about and have contact with older people.

Design and methods

In stage one of the project, questionnaires and video studies were used with the full sample. The methods were modified for the old people, some of whom required help to write answers to questions. In stage two, field studies were carried out in a small number of primary health care teams, using a Prompt List for assessment, developed from the video studies. Details of stage two are available in the full report.[6]

Video studies

During exploratory work, the researchers first examined their own styles and methods of assessing old people at home by video-recording interviews with elderly ladies with multiple disabilities. These videos provided one of the principal study methods.

A three-and-a-half minute excerpt of an interview with an elderly lady with mobility problems was selected and shown to all study participants, including the old people. First, the scene was set by giving written information:

> 'The doctor on duty the previous night says he has seen Mrs C., an eighty-four year old widow, who has fallen. Fortunately, there is no serious injury. The doctor asks you to visit her. She is not previously known to you.'

On the video, Mrs C. was shown seated in a low armchair. She struggled to rise from it and walked across the room with a limp, using her stick and the furniture for support. She sat down heavily into a higher chair by the window and began to discuss her past and current health and home circumstances.

A series of questions was then posed to which written and time-limited responses were invited:

> Q.1. What have you seen and heard of significance? List your observations.

> Q.2. What actual and potential problems do you think Mrs C. has? List the problems.

> Q.3. At the end of your interview, what areas of assessment would you wish to have covered?

Observations and problems

Overall, many observations and problems were defined on the basis of a video stimulus lasting only three and a half minutes; there were 170 different responses.

There were surprising differences in the ways in which Mrs C. and her surroundings were perceived. For example, she was variously described as cheerful, depressed, anxious, stubborn, bored, lonely, withdrawn, dogmatic, proud, realistic, apathetic and having a sense of humour. She was regarded as neat, tidy and well dressed but also unkempt. Her room was described as cluttered and uncluttered and the house as suitable and unsuitable. Individual professionals perceived this lady and her circumstances in quite different and sometimes opposing ways.

There was within-group and between-group consensus about certain categories of observations and problems; however, there were also differences in detail which reflected different professional perspectives. For example, the opening scene in which Mrs C. tried to rise with difficulty from the low chair was interpreted by a general practitioner as a problem of arthritic hips, by a health visitor student as a problem of too low a chair, and by a physiotherapy student as a problem of leverage and poor hand function.

A clear focus for problem definition was not always evident for each group. However, social work students consistently commented about Mrs C.'s mood, feelings and attitudes, the contact of her family and the support available from them. The occupational therapy students noted possible problems with dressing, shopping, cooking and home safety, and physiotherapy students gave the most detail about balance, movement, the risks of falling, transferring from bed, chairs and toilet, hand function and grip strength.

Scope and content of assessment

There were 235 different responses which fell into forty-six categories. The scope of assessment was therefore wide, and there was considerable overlap between groups of participants with almost every category mentioned by each group. It was encouraging to find that the range of content of assessment was very similar for the old people; forty-two of the forty-six categories were mentioned by them. The scope and content are summarised on the Prompt List (Figure 1).

There were, however, major and worrying gaps overall in key areas of assessment:

feet	*memory and orientation*
continence	*attitudes and feelings of carers*
hearing	*medication*
sleep	*bereavement*
security and telephone	*teeth*

On paper, individual responses to the questions varied widely from a few words to a tightly-packed and well-structured page of assessment categories and detail within categories. Some participants had a clear and detailed framework of assessment in their heads, others did not.

The starting point or focus of assessment provided another interesting area of difference in the pattern of responses on paper. For example, the occupational therapy and physiotherapy students started with mobility and extrapolated from it to other areas of assessment. The social work students started by wishing to enquire about the old lady's attitudes, views and feelings about her own health, her housing, her wish and need for help, and about the future. They also wished to assess the views of the old lady's relatives and helpers; they then moved on to practical prob-

Figure 1 - Prompt List for Health Assessment of the Elderly

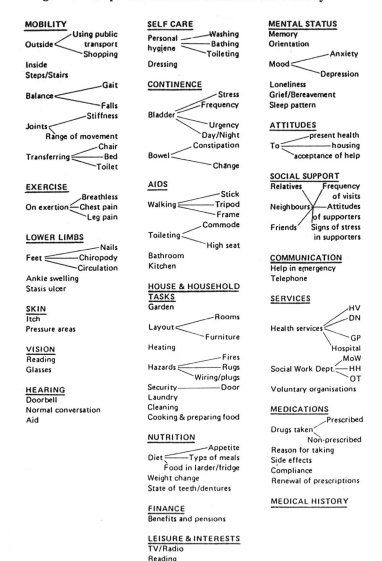

MOBILITY
Outside — Using public transport / Shopping
Inside
Steps/Stairs
Balance — Gait / Falls
Joints — Stiffness
Range of movement
Transferring — Chair / Bed / Toilet

EXERCISE
On exertion — Breathless / Chest pain / Leg pain

LOWER LIMBS
Feet — Nails / Chiropody / Circulation
Ankle swelling
Stasis ulcer

SKIN
Itch
Pressure areas

VISION
Reading
Glasses

HEARING
Doorbell
Normal conversation
Aid

SELF CARE
Personal hygiene — Washing / Bathing / Toileting
Dressing

CONTINENCE
Bladder — Stress / Frequency / Urgency / Day/Night
Bowel — Constipation / Change

AIDS
Walking — Stick / Tripod / Frame
Toileting — Commode / High seat
Bathroom
Kitchen

HOUSE & HOUSEHOLD TASKS
Garden
Layout — Rooms / Furniture
Heating
Hazards — Fires / Rugs / Wiring/plugs
Security — Door
Laundry
Cleaning
Cooking & preparing food

NUTRITION
Diet — Appetite / Type of meals / Food in larder/fridge
Weight change
State of teeth/dentures

FINANCE
Benefits and pensions

LEISURE & INTERESTS
TV/Radio
Reading
Pets
Outings
Smoking and alcohol

MENTAL STATUS
Memory
Orientation
Mood — Anxiety / Depression
Loneliness
Grief/Bereavement
Sleep pattern

ATTITUDES
To — present health / housing / acceptance of help

SOCIAL SUPPORT
Relatives / Frequency of visits
Neighbours — Attitudes of supporters
Friends / Signs of stress in supporters

COMMUNICATION
Help in emergency
Telephone

SERVICES
Health services — HV / DN / GP / Hospital
Social Work Dept. — MoW / HH / OT
Voluntary organisations

MEDICATIONS
Drugs taken — Prescribed / Non-prescribed
Reason for taking
Side effects
Compliance
Renewal of prescriptions

MEDICAL HISTORY

From: BUCKLEY E. G. and RUNCIMAN P. J. 1985 Health Assessment of the Elderly at Home University of Edinburgh.

lems associated with mobility and environment. The health visitor students demonstrated no clear focus or starting point.

Luker[10] suggests that health visitors may have difficulty working with old people because they lack a framework for health assessment of the elderly. This study suggests, however, that some student and experienced health visitors do have a clear and well-developed framework for assessment, but that health visitors as a group lack a consistent focus or framework pattern for assessment.

It could be argued that one of the potential strengths of health visitors in health assessment of old people is their breadth of perspective and that the lack of a consistent pattern does not matter. It may be appropriate to vary the starting point and route through an assessment interview according to the problems and cues presented, the observations made and the dynamics of the interaction with the old person. Sensitive participation in and 'control' of an interview requires considerable knowledge and skill.

These findings support Rowlings'[11] contention that

'all staff concerned with assessment interviews should be competent at interviewing and not just at obtaining information.'

Care provision

A final set of questions was designed to explore care provision for the elderly lady on the trigger video. Additional information was given to develop the scenario and participants were asked:

'Should this lady be visited? If so, by whom, for what reasons and how frequently?'

It was found that every group felt they had a contribution to make to her assessment and care, and there was considerable overlap of functions. The perception of the role of other professionals was narrower than the perception of one's own role and there was marked role stereotyping. It was felt that the old lady should be visited from as often as daily to as seldom as six monthly.

The impact of education and training

Health visitor and district nurse students participated in the video studies twice, the first occasion being near the beginning of their course, the second after a six month interval and following some practice experience and theoretical input on the elderly. Overall, it seemed that their education and training had little positive impact and it could be argued that this is not surprising as these groups did not receive *specific* guidance for this part of their work. However, there was evidence from the video responses of the district nurse students late in training that they had adopted a particular theoretical framework to assessment of health needs during their course and that this had become a barrier to detailed consideration of an individual's health needs.

Views and feelings about visiting old people

Included in a questionnaire were two questions which related to the second aim of the study:

- Health professionals have different views and feelings about working with older people. How do you feel about visiting the elderly at home?
- Are there any particular experiences which have influenced your views about visiting the elderly - experiences during training at work, with friends or relatives...?

Visiting elderly people was often described as rewarding, worthwhile and satisfying. But it could also be frustrating and depressing and some participants felt angry and disillusioned about this part of their work. Overall, responses were more often positive than negative; but many remarks were qualified, indicating a considerable amount of ambivalence.

It is important to acknowledge that such a range and depth of feelings may exist, as it became clear that feelings influenced the willingness and ability of participants to work in this area of care.

Four main themes emerged. Comments have been selected from the student groups to illustrate each theme.

1. Priorities and preferences

General practitioner trainees, district nurse, health visitor and social work students all commented about the competing claims upon their time.

A general practitioner trainee remarked that visiting and assessing elderly people could be low priority and 'temporarily put off' in favour of 'more urgent calls'; 'too much home visiting chokes the visit book and leaves less time for the people who are ill and those who need support on a short-term basis.'

A social work student suggested that in her training the elderly were considered 'worthy of equal respect' but in reality there was 'a feeling in social work still that work with the elderly has low status; that the elderly do not warrant the same intervention and attention as other groups, for example, children.'

The work of district nurses is predominantly with old people and their views were rather different; some district nurse students wished to have more involvement with younger age groups. Also, student and experienced district nurses wished to have more time to 'visit the well elderly with the emphasis on prevention rather than curative nursing.'

The dilemma for health visitors reflected the traditional orientation towards work with the under fives and young families. It seemed that some health visitors neither wished nor expected to work with old people.

'My own personal interest is with children ... For me, the priority should be given to the young as they are the elderly of tomorrow.' *(Student HV)*

'I feel it is locking the stable door after the horse is gone ... Efforts should be started at pre-retiral age. You are unlikely to influence elderly people greatly at their stage of life as they are set in their ways.' *(Student HV)*

Primary and secondary prevention were felt to merit more attention than tertiary prevention. However, the suggestion that work with old people is necessarily orientated towards tertiary prevention, and that old people are 'set in their ways' should be debated. It could be argued that many health promotion and disease prevention activities are possible even where disability is established. It also seemed to the researchers, that many of the 'young' and 'middle aged' participants in the study were as set, or more set, in their ways than the old people captured on video!

The following remark of an occupational therapy student was echoed by social work students:

'Mixed feelings ... some visits to elderly people are interesting and enjoyable and others are horrendous - when the person has been very incontinent. On the whole, I don't particularly enjoy visiting the elderly at home but think it necessary.' *(Student OT)*

This remark is a thought-provoking reminder to the core team of health visitors, district nurses and general practitioners who, over their years of professional experience, may have become accustomed to the often distressing circumstances of some old people, particularly in relation to dementia, incontinence and poor or dirty home conditions. It seems that within the team, there may be at times a lack of awareness of the feelings of colleagues and failure to offer support to students and trainees.

2. Skills and training

> 'I feel a bit inadequate at present in assessing the needs of the elderly in view of my lack of formal training in this discipline.' *(Trainee GP)*

> 'I do not mind visiting the elderly, but find it difficult sometimes to know what to do once I am there if it is not an acute problem.' *(Trainee GP)*

Health assessment was regarded by participants in all groups as a vague and difficult activity. Two problems in particular were experienced. Assessment of older people could be 'time consuming' and 'lengthy', and there were 'sensitive' or 'delicate' areas about which it was difficult to enquire and which old people might be reluctant to discuss; for example, continence and finance.

Several questions emerge from these problems:

- Is the professional clear about the purpose and scope of assessment?

- Is the old person clear about the purpose of the visit? It was felt that when clients perceived an assessment visit as a social call, the professional could be swept along on a conversational tide.

- Is the interviewer able to make appropriate observations, to use direct but tactful questions about 'sensitive' areas, and to check the reliability of observations made and information obtained?

- Is time available, or other personnel available, for follow-up visits? A social work student remarked that 'mood and behaviour fluctuate and one visit may not be enough.' Health visitors felt that repeated visits were important for several reasons. Many older people were unsure at first about who the health visitor was, where she came from and what she did. The health visitors also felt that 'relationship making' was 'an investment for the future.' It did seem, however, that remarks such as 'we need to spend time forming a relationship' and 'we only get a true picture after several visits' might have masked basic problems with interviewing skills.

3. Work organisation and the team

There were two main problem areas.

First, roles and relationships. Students were clearly aware of the tensions within teams; teamwork seemed to be more myth than reality:

> 'I would have liked the health visitor to work with the elderly but our relationship and communication are far from ideal.' *(GP)*

'I feel helpless because of the GP's attitude. I would find it more rewarding if the GP participated in discussion.' *(HV)*

There was also anxiety about 'duplication of visiting'. Several professionals could be knocking on the same door, each one failing to get in touch with the others involved. Lack of knowledge of respective roles was thought to be one cause of the problem, but lack of thought, discussion and coordination were also evident.

'I am worried about the number of disciplines that visit an elderly person during a crisis period ... Very often this causes distress, confusion and a reluctance to accept services. Perhaps an integrated, coordinated approach would be more acceptable.' *(Home Care Organiser)*

Second, resources and services:

'I feel useless if the services required are not available. Identifying need without resources is disheartening.' *(Student HV)*

Each group, except the general practitioner trainees, made some comment reflecting 'frustration', 'bitterness' and a sense of 'helplessness' because of 'lack of back-up' from health and social services. The GP trainees may not have voiced such frustration because most of their experience had been in the episodic management of illness rather than in continuing contact with older people with chronic problems.

4. Feelings and rights of the elderly

Within all groups there was evidence of sensitivity to the feelings and rights of old people.

'With frail, sometimes confused elderly, I feel that the roles of relatives, friends, neighbours, home helps, ministers, etc. are all very difficult to sort out. I am concerned about the elderly person's rights in all this.' *(Student SW)*

It was suggested that at times, old people need considerable strength to withstand the often uncoordinated onslaught of the many professionals who visit to 'offer help'.

Overall, old people were regarded as welcoming and appreciative of assessment and it was felt that they enjoyed the company and contact with visitors. However, it was acknowledged that some distrusted 'interference' and resented 'prying'. Many had considerable pride, were fiercely independent and reluctant to 'accept charity'. Others felt that it was their right to have the GP 'keep an eye on them'.

It was noted that whereas some old people 'didn't like to be a bother', others welcomed 'being of interest'. Some actively sought help for their difficulties and disabilities while others felt 'it's just old age', 'nothing can be done' and 'there's always somebody worse off than me'.

It was recognised that an old person and a health professional might not share priorities and points of view and this could be 'exasperating', but it was acknowledged that old people should have 'every right to refuse help' and 'could choose to live with risks.'

Despite the frustrations inherent in this part of their work, it was striking that all groups commented about the rewards of working with old people.

Recommendations

The health problems of the elderly can appear to be so large that they paralyze action. The educational recommendations which can be made from this study, however, suggest ways in which student and experienced workers could be helped to learn about and deal more effectively with assessment of the health of old people at home.

The first essential is that responsible institutions acknowledge the need for specific education and training for health assessment of old people. Education should be based on reality. Exploration of theories, models and concepts of ageing is of value but should not be a substitute for developing skills in interviewing old people and for exploring ways of helping them and their carers with practical problems.

The use of short excerpts of video recordings of real interviews is a powerful teaching method which enables learning to be focussed, structured and based in reality. It is also a technique which facilitates the discussion of emotive ethical issues.

The prompt list, created from the responses of the participants in the study, has been found to be useful as a framework for teaching and as a framework for health assessment in practice.

In recent years there have been many imaginative developments in case finding and screening of the elderly in Britain and these have been reviewed fully in an occasional paper of the Royal College of General Practitioners.[12] Student and experienced health care workers should know about and be encouraged to explore such developments.

This study has confirmed that many professional groups wish to be involved in health assessment of old people, that roles of different members of the care team overlap and that educational activities whenever possible should be multidisciplinary. Shared learning, however, has been slow to develop and difficult to achieve at all levels in Britain. At basic and post-basic levels, students from different disciplines seldom learn together although the relevant professional bodies have made recommendations and supported joint educational initiatives. In continuing education, there is an urgent need for educational activities to become part of the day-to-day functioning of the team.

Reasons for delay in developing shared learning are not hard to find and Jones[13] has suggested that the problems are both organisational and attitudinal: issues of structures and funding as well as priorities and commitment need to be addressed. It would seem that the development of shared learning remains as one of the major challenges for the latter part of this century.

References

1. Schrock, R. 'Elderly People in Contemporary Society'. In Cormack, D. (ed.) *Geriatric Nursing. A Conceptual Approach*. Blackwell Scientific Publications, Oxford, 1985.

2. Rowlings, C. 'Practice in Field Care'. In Lishman, J. (ed.) *Developing Services for the Elderly* (2nd Edition). Research Highlights, No.3. Kogan Page, London, 1985.

3. McClymont, M. et al. *Health Visiting and the Elderly*. Churchill Livingstone, Edinburgh, 1986.

4. Ross, F. 'District Nursing' *Recent Advances in Nursing: Community Nursing*. 15, 1987, 132-160.

5. Beth Johnson Foundation. 'The Senior Health Shop' *Update*. 5, 1, Spring/Summer, 1987.

6. Buckley, E.G., and Runciman, P.J. *Health Assessment of the Elderly at Home*. University of Edinburgh, 1985.

7. Hudson, B. 'Jack of All Trades?' *Health and Social Service Journal*. 88, 4580, 1978, 251.

8. Day, L. 'Health Visiting and the Elderly in the 1980's - Do We Care Enough?' *Health Visitor*. 54, 12, 1981, 538-539.

9. Rowlings, C. *Social Work with Elderly People*. George Allen and Unwin, London, 1981.

10. Luker, K. *Evaluating Health Visiting Practice*. Royal College of Nursing, London, 1982.

11. Rowlings, C. op. cit. 1981, p.75.

12. Taylor, R.C., and Buckley, E.G. *Preventive Care of the Elderly: A Review of Current Developments*. Occasional paper 35, The Royal College of General Practitioners, London, 1987.

13. Jones, R. *Working Together - Learning Together*. Occasional paper 33, The Royal College of General Practitioners, London, 1986.

Acknowledgements

The partnership of Dr. Graham Buckley during the research is acknowledged. Dr. Buckley is a General Practitioner at Livingston, West Lothian, and Editor of the *Journal of the Royal College of General Practitioners*.

Professional Ideology or Organisational Tribalism? The Health Service-Social Work Divide

Gillian Dalley

The promotion of 'teamwork' as a means of providing better and more integrated services to the clients of health and social service agencies has a history, some would say, dating as far back as the 1920s with the publication of the Dawson report on the future provision of medical and allied services.[1] That report argued for the development of health centres as the way forward in providing an integrated system of primary care; it described a network of what it referred to as primary and secondary health centres with doctors, dentists, pharmacists, nurses, midwives and health visitors all working collaboratively from the primary health centres to provide a service to local populations.

The concept of the primary health care team itself began to emerge more concretely during the 1960s. The Harding report on the primary health care team published in 1981[2] reviews its development. It cites a report from the Standing Medical Advisory Committee of the Central Health Services Council in 1963 as recommending that 'fieldworkers such as the nurse, midwife and health visitor should be attached to individual (GP) practices.' A conference in 1969 on the work of the team in family health care sponsored jointly by the Health Visitors Association, the National Association of State Enrolled Nurses, the Queen's Institute of District Nurses, the Royal Colleges of General Practitioners, of Midwives, and of Nurses, and the Society of Medical Officers of Health spent two days exploring the role of the team and the part it should play in the future development of primary health care. The 1970s saw many more workshops, seminars and conferences convened to promote the team concept and to discuss the need for inter-professional training as a means of establishing an appropriate environment for the initiation of teamworking.

Teamwork was advocated not only for those working within the health service; it was seen as a means of achieving greater collaboration *between* agencies. The Seebohm report published in 1968[3] and primarily concerned with recommending the establishment of generic social services departments, also discussed the importance of establishing collaborative relationships with the primary care services and considered how this could be achieved through teamwork:

'We regard teamwork between general practitioners and the social services as vital. It is one of our main objectives and the likelihood of promoting it is a test we would like to see applied to our proposals for a social service department' (i.e. the centrepiece of the report).

Central government policy has for a long time accepted the stream of recommendations about teamwork coming from this variety of reports. The 1974 Annual Report of the DHSS[4] pronounced one of its aims as being the creation of

'primary health care teams in which general medical practitioners, home nurses, health visitors and in some cases social workers and dentists, work together as an inter-disciplinary team, thus facilitating co-ordination and mutual support in the planning and delivery of care.'

Other policy documents produced during the 1970s also stressed the importance of teamworking. The 1976 'Priorities' document[5] set out as one of its main objectives

'to encourage the development of primary health care teams in order to improve preventive and curative services in the community ..., to allow for the increased workload which will result from the greater number of old people ... (and) reduce demands on the acute hospital services.'

It saw the continued growth of health centres as facilitating the development of teamwork.

Over a decade later, the White Paper on primary care published in 1987,[6] reaffirmed the importance that central government placed on the concept of the primary health care team:

'the services provided by nurses, midwives and health visitors (along with GPs) are an important part of the totality of primary health care. Primary care is at its best when provided by a range of professional staff, working together as members of a primary health care team ... the Government attaches considerable importance to the strengthening of the primary health care team.'

Most recently, the need for effective teamworking in the provision of co-ordinated services has been stressed by the report of the Butler-Sloss inquiry into child abuse in Cleveland.[7] It recommended the establishment of multi-disciplinary teams with the

'intention to foster teamwork and co-ordination of activity without undermining primary professional responsibility or agency function.'

The team, then, has been and still is seen by policy-makers and planners as the main instrument for achieving collaborative relationships between professions and between agencies in the provision and delivery of integrated care.

But just as central government was making a commitment to the concept of the team and to teamworking, reports from practitioners and from academic research began to demonstrate the problems arising from attempts to initiate teamworking. Evidence taken by the Harding committee and cited in the report[2] from practitioners and managers in the field saw problems arising from three different sources: one was to do with poor accommodation and lack of resources which imposed too great a burden on health visiting and district nursing staff; another was the structural problem - GPs were independent contractors while nursing staff were part of the health authority management structure; the third was the difference in outlook between the different professional groups involved and the lack of understanding of each other's roles and orientations that this involved.

This latter difficulty is one which has been considered by a number of academic writers. Strauss, Schatzman, Bucher, Ehrlich and Sabshin[8] in a study of psychiatric institutions concluded that ideology affected the organisation of care and treatment especially in relation to the division of labour; they used the concept of 'operational philosophies' to account for the way in which specific ideologies are put into practice in daily action. The importance of professional ideology was also stressed by Marx,[9] who recognised that different professional groupings brought different ideologies to bear within the same arena, creating tensions and conflictual relationships. Mauksch[10] described how ideologies sometimes complement each other but frequently compete in intra-institutional negotiations. Smith, in a study of social workers and the operation of the children's panel system in Scotland,[11] introduced the concept of the 'situated account' to describe the manner in which professional ideologies - which related to the overarching, more abstract level of thought - were modified to provide a rationale for everyday action. Both he and Goldie[12] suggested that there might be a number of ideologies operating within a single profession.

Much has been written specifically on the workings (and failings) of 'the team' in the health and social services worlds - see, for example, Lonsdale, Webb and Briggs[13] and Bruce[14] - often using the concept of ideology as an explanatory factor in describing why teams often do not work well. Writing about the relationship between health visitors and social workers, Dingwall[15] suggested that differences in attitudes and beliefs had created a climate of hostility which had become self-fulfilling. Huntington, in a study of social work and general practice,[16] describes the two 'occupational cultures' which each of the professional groups inhabits and which inhibit practitioners from developing collaborative working relationships. More recently, a study of collaborative relationships in the primary health care setting by Cartlidge, Bond and Gregson[17] concludes that levels of collaboration are low.

The view, then, is widely held that differences in the belief systems and attitude sets of the various professional groups inhibits co-operation. The medical practitioner is seen to be held deep in the grip of the 'medical model'; the social worker cleaves to a psycho-social perspective on the world which contests the individualised, disease centred medical view. Nurses, of all sorts, are trapped in a deferential relationship with doctors which they resent but from which they cannot escape. This, of course, caricatures the position to a certain degree but much of the evidence available points towards this interpretation.

The research evidence

In research conducted by the present writer examining professional attitudes to a number of policy issues - concerning, in particular, community care and policies for the priority groups - patterns of views which were distinctive of particular professional groups certainly emerged. Further, many instances of difficulties in inter-professional working were also described. Two hundred and thirty-six individuals were interviewed, in three Scottish locations; they were drawn from a wide variety of professional groupings within the health and social services - hospital consultants, GPs, health visitors, district nurses, ward sisters, NHS managers, basic grade social workers and social work managers of all levels.

Inter-professional working

The most numerous instances of incompatibility in working together arose between GPs and social workers; but there were many other difficulties recorded, between social workers and health visitors, between health visitors and GPs, between GPs and hospital consultants and between hospital based social workers and consultants. Difficulties were expressed in both the practical terms of organisational and structural issues and the abstract terms of orientation and attitudes. For instance, one GP found difficulties in working with social workers because of the way their work was organised:

'I think again one of the difficulties is that the way the social work teams are arranged - one of them has a particular responsibility for the elderly, one for the handicapped, one for children, so that again tends to cut across what we do'.

Another GP referred to the competition between medicine and social work in the definition of problems:

> 'doctors and social workers - again you vie for whether a problem is a social or a medical problem ... to establish precedence there'.

In the case of a district nurse, difficulties in working with both GPs and social workers were described:

> 'I feel it very much ... it's very frustrating ... You're a buffer in the fact that you've got the doctor you liaise with, she comes back and says I want this that and the other, you go to the social work department and get nothing from them. And I feel, well, you know, I thought it was teamwork and here's me going in, and I just felt nothing was being done'.

Another district nurse expressed resentment of some GPs:

> 'I think some GPs will tend to, what shall I say, throw all the dregs of the day at you ... if the GP is not very helpful at, say, getting the geriatrician out, then you're left with it to do'.

In the case of social workers, hostility towards health visitors was sometimes expressed by them in terms of differences in fundamental attitudes:

> 'Yes, I think there is a difference between our attitudes certainly, from our experience with health visitors. And their whole training has been to take a person into care and to - in many ways take away their rights, I suppose - and our training leans to the opposite point of view almost and I think there is some kind of friction in our attitudes on many points'.

Similar hostility was felt by some social workers towards GPs:

> 'I think that there certainly is a lack of understanding by a large number of GPs of the social work role. It's a suspicion and it's also at its worst (because they think) that if they do begin to develop a relationship then there's a floodgate opening ... that's again to do with the structure and the pressure they can be under as much as any real recalcitrance'.

Evidence such as this, then, demonstrates a widespread sense of discontent with regard to the success of inter-professional working. Explanations of the failure to collaborate successfully is put down both to structural difficulties - the way the services operate, differences in organisation, lack of understanding about the pressures under which colleagues in different professions have to work and so on - and to differences in approach and orientation. Just as academic analysts have identified 'professional ideology' as a barrier to co-operation, so practitioners recognise the same constraints. A social worker, talking about health visitors, for example, described them as adopting a medical view of old people's needs for care in contrast to their (social work) views:

'these people (old people) don't want - they want to go back to their independence - it's the health visitor's anxiety coming through, and not the person's, you know the old folk. And that is unethical ... And very often they see it purely from a medical point of view and not - they don't consider the emotional stress'.

A senior social worker, who led a team working exclusively in a primary care setting, in a health centre with attachments to a number of group practices, expressed her disappointment at their failure to establish successful inter-professional working:

'I have felt disappointed in the level of co-ordination - you know, I feel that things should be better co-ordinated in a primary care team, and that patient management ought to be optimum - but I mean, dreadful things happen - and people fall between, even where there's a nurse, a health visitor, a doctor and a social worker. And everybody is assuming that somebody else is doing it ... I think professional orientation (causes it). Partly the problem is that health visitors and nurses feel they can do nothing without asking the doctor'.

The role of professional ideology

Practitioners may *believe* and report that they view things differently from those in other professional groups; it is important from an analytical standpoint, however, to investigate how far such ideological cleavages exist in reality. The interview study covered a wide range of topics concerning both the politico-moral domain (questions, for example, about the balance of social responsibility for the care of dependent people, as between family and state; the role of voluntarism in welfare) and the practical issues of resource allocation for the priority groups (covering, for example, the relationship between institutional and community care; the degree to which resources should be invested in prevention or withdrawn from the acute sector).

When responses to the politico-moral issues are examined, it is clear that significant differences between professional groups emerge. Most striking was the contrast between GPs and many of the other groups in respect of their views about the question of responsibility. More than three quarters of GPs interviewed felt that it was predominantly the responsibility of families to care for dependent members, as opposed to just over a third of basic grade social workers and half of health visitors. In contrast, almost two thirds of social workers felt it was a matter of state respon-

the health visitors and social work and NHS managers. District nurses were more like GPs though less overwhelmingly supportive of the 'family responsibility' position.

The following remarks of one GP were characteristic of many:

'Morally it should be the family (taking responsibility) but then we're not living in a very moral age. And the families just don't want to know - the hard fact is that people really don't want to have this burden'.

Another GP voiced similar views:

'I would like to see much more family responsibility but modern society has drifted away from it and there's nothing really that medical people can do about it unless the society as a whole accepts the need for, morally accepts the need for care by the family'.

A majority of district nurses mirrored this view:

'I see it in this country the way we run things, then I see it's got to be the family has the prime responsibility often the family should and could help a lot more - because it's their folks, they should have a responsibility to their own people'.

Social workers, on the other hand, viewed things rather differently:

'Well I think we live in a society which has admitted by stating it's a democracy ... that the community is responsible for the community ... well, actually, well the state, I think I have to say the community and the state'.

and

'It comes back to the question of what is community care. You know, because can the community care for the family as a whole? Maybe the family needs to be cared for by the community and that would include any relatives with particular problems. I certainly, I think, I don't think I would go along with the argument that the family ought to care and that's all there is to it ... no, I think certainly the state ought to care ... has a responsibility to see that ... the dependency groups, to see that they are being cared for'.

Health visitors spoke in a similar vein:

'I have great sympathy for relatives. I think it should be a state responsibility. Um, it would be nice to see relatives getting more involved with the elderly - er - but it can be very difficult for them. They can be made to feel very guilty if they don't look after their relatives'.

Perceptions about the public tended to match views about the issue of responsibility. Those who believed it was a family responsibility to care tended also to believe that the public in general was reluctant to care and that too much was expected of professionally provided services. A number of GPs were very judgemental in their views of the public:

'I would say the majority (of the public) opt out. Fewer and fewer folk are going to upset their own lives at all to cope with their own relatives. I think they're being selfish and not accepting of the position'.

and

'To get a family to care for an elderly relative they have to be, have affection for that relative, they have to understand the problems, they have to care about people in general and ... they don't. That's a bit general, but people are too involved with what they want to get out of life ... I think they should take a greater responsibility'.

and

'I do blame the old people themselves ... because they voted for this system ... and they have done nothing to change it ... they have sat expecting me and the nurse and everybody else to supply what they want ... until they die. I do blame them and ... as a GP what I do notice is that the old people of 70 and 80 today are not the same as old people when I started out ... they're two different breeds ... the present lot expect to be kept as 60 year olds forever'.

But those who saw a greater responsibility lying with the state, tended also at the same time to be less judgemental of the public. They were more ready to see the strain and stress that is often involved in caring for a dependent relative and felt that the public had the right to expect more from the services. A social worker said:

'I think they (the public) should expect more if they want it ... I think they are willing (to care) in the sense that they want to but sometimes - it's usually the partner you know, if it's something like the mother's mother then it's usually the husband so they have torn loyalties between the two'.

and another social worker:

'I find the majority of them are (willing to care), it's surprising the amount of wives, spouses, that accept the nature of their spouse's illness - mental or whatever ... and stand by them'.

Some health visitors felt similarly:

'I don't think so (that people expect too much of the services), I feel that the people I've come across who have some quite hard jobs with elderly relatives, I think actually sometimes put up with quite a lot more than perhaps I would expect to myself ... yes, I think the majority of them are (willing to care). I mean, saying that, I have come across people who just don't want to know at all. But again, few and far between'.

Fewer district nurses were so sympathetic although a number were:

'There's always the minority that'll always want more but to be truthful the majority of patients are very grateful, they think they're getting a lot ... there's always the majority we feel that are willing to take responsibility ... as long as they're getting that wee bit of support from the backup services'.

Most were more sceptical about the public though:

'they're liable to say "Oh get the nurse in, you should have a nurse to do that". I think people become selfish - they don't realise just how many dependent people there are ... Nowadays a number of them are not (prepared to care) - people are too busy with their own lives now'.

Ideology can be defined as a patterning of beliefs and values relating to a view of the ordering of the world at relatively high levels of abstraction; *professional* ideology is that part of wider ideology which underpins world views insofar as they relate to professional practice. The views expressed here about the politico-moral issues of social responsibility, it is argued, fall into this category. On the evidence derived from the interview study, it seems clear that ideological differences emerge on these issues between some groups of 'front-line' practitioners located in both the health and social services. At one extreme are the GPs who hold strong and judgemental views about the moral responsibility of families to care; at the other extreme are social workers who have a more open view about the moral position: the state has an underlying responsibility, although families also have a role. They tend not to 'judge' the public by perceiving it as morally deficient in failing to accept responsibility. Located somewhere midway between the two are health visitors and district nurses.

Force of circumstance: the conditioning of everyday action

The investigation of attitudes in the politico-moral domain reveals the existence of clear ideological differences between professional groups. This confirms the findings of other research studies and it also confirms the views of practitioners themselves; as discussed above, they tend to account for failures in inter-professional working in terms of fundamental differences in attitudes.

But further investigation of front-line workers' attitudes demonstrates a degree of *similarity* in views on some issues. This is often most clearly revealed when their views are set against the views of other categories of respondents - managers and hospital based staff, for example. Managers in both the health and social services, for example, frequently showed a greater empathy for the public than the community-based front-line practitioners who, in fact, had the greatest contact with them. In spite of the ideological contrasts between, say, general practitioners and social workers, or health visitors and social workers, these were frequently cross-cut by contrasts between all of them on the one hand and managers, removed from the field, on the other.

Thus managers could express positive feelings towards the public untempered by direct knowledge of the reality of the circumstances - both the difficulties faced by, and created by, the public and the heavy strain placed on some field staff by those difficulties. Field staff were often torn between feeling sympathy for their clients but also frustrated and pressured by them. A sector administrator, for example, recognised that he did not have direct experience of the problem.

'As I say, not coming directly in contact with a lot of them, but I do obviously speak a lot to nursing officers and medical people ... but you do hear of families doing this and that ... and who do realise that they have a role to play'.

This respondent thought highly of the public but tended to be critical of some practitioners. He recounted a case where a family had requested the use of a particular sort of bed - in his view, legitimately - but the nurse involved had felt them to be too demanding; he was critical of GPs, suggesting that they did too little for dependent people:

'I think it's a pity. I think the GP was and should be somebody who is held in high esteem by the population. And I think services provided by us in the community would seem so much better if the GP was generally accepted as being the man that they admired and would come at a call. I know that they've got limited resources, that they've got limited time, but there is no doubt that the GP of today does not put the work into the job or the time'.

In contrast, however, were the views of practitioners who held more jaundiced views of the public. A health visitor, for example, said:

'I think it's because the great wave of unemployment and whatnot has tended - I'm talking about the people in this area, not about the people outwith it, but in this area the dependency on state aid is vast and they do an awful lot of taking and not a lot of giving, I'm afraid ... They don't want to take responsibility for themselves. Not here. My caseload is made up of people who have not taken responsibility for their own lives, therefore that's why they run into social problems, because they don't think'.

And yet this was a respondent who believed firmly that the state was responsible for providing care and support to those who were dependent.

In respect of issues which were the direct concern of managers and more removed from field staff - issues of resource allocation and strategic policy, for example - front-line practitioners tended to be able to offer answers directly, while managers responded in a much more circumscribed way. For them, the dilemmas were real, for practitioners, the problem of decision-making in these matters was hypothetical and therefore less charged with complexity. On the question of support for central government's priority policies (favouring the priority groups over the acute sector), front-line practitioners were more firmly in support than their managers who, while coming out in support, were much more equivocal in their responses. An NHS manager, for example, supported the policies in principle:

'Yes, I'd agree with that policy provided that you have to have - you still have to have acute medical, sufficient acute medical services so that they can cope with the needs of the community ... I mean, it's said in Glasgow that there are too many acute beds, too many acute medical wards and that this should be run down a bit to make priority for these dependency groups. All I know is that every winter, it's the same story. Every hospital has difficulty in finding a bed to take people into'.

But a front-line worker, a social worker, answered much more directly:

'Yes, I think we have a responsibility to cater for the disabled ... the elderly, the chronically sick, the people who do require additional support and services ... Old age is something that happens, chronic, mental or physical disability, these are things over which people have very marginal control ... we should spend a good percentage of our time concentrating on these people ... Mine happens to be a very personalised view because I work in this field'.

The evidence seems to suggest, then, that although professional ideology is a strong and binding influence in contributing to group identity, the factor of circumstances is also at work, cutting across ideological ties. The experience of working at the front-line, at the interface between the public as clients and the services, confers a commonality of attitudes about certain issues amongst practitioners, just as the responsibility of managerial decision-making binds managers together in their views irrespective of their agency or professional background.

Tribal ties: beliefs or allegiances?

Individuals belonging to the same professional group exhibit many attitudes in common especially, as has been discussed, at the ideological level. Similarly, individuals working under common circumstances, in the same or parallel structural positions, hold certain views in common - cutting across professional boundaries. But further examination of responses shows yet another dimension; it relates to respondents' perceptions about themselves, their attitudes and about others.

Objectively, it is fair to say that there are real problems related to different ideological views which inhibit inter-professional co-operation, and the individuals involved recognise this. Equally, there are many common experiences and attitudes which link these same individuals. But as important, are their *perceptions* that they are different and in some sense in opposition. The strength of what Huntington[16] calls occupational culture, or what here could well be called corporate identity or *organisational* culture, fuels whatever cleavages or bondings already exist. Huntington tends to see professional ideology as a part of occupational culture; it is perhaps more helpful to separate them as constructs. Professional ideology relates to particular sets of values and moral attitudes, generally acquired implicitly over time through the training and induction processes of professional qualification; organisational culture is a means of drawing explicit boundaries around a group, imbuing the group with a view about itself that proclaims its distinctiveness as being characterised by particular behaviours and attitudes (whether or not it really is distinctive). It is the certainty that it is, and the allegiance to the group which that stimulates, that is significant - hence the label 'tribalism'.

In some instances, professional ideology and organisational culture (or tribalism) may act to reinforce each other; the profession may also be the group. This is perhaps true of social work since it tends to be a single profession department (although that is to ignore the differences which are known to exist between levels of qualification and spheres of work - CQSW/CSS; casework/residential care work, for example). In the case of the health service, there are a number of professional groupings located within the larger organisational space - often with clearly articulated differences in ideology. But those professional groupings tend to coalesce when set against another organisation or agency - such as a social services or social work department. The cleavage then becomes an inter-agency rather than an inter-professional one: one of culture rather than of ideology.

Evidence for this proposition can be found in the interview study. Differences emerged between members of social work departments on the one hand and members (of several professional groupings) of the health service on the other, irrespective of the similarity of many of their views. On occasion, the opposite agency and its members might be ascribed certain views which they did not in fact hold. The issue of community care versus institutional care is a good example of how the members of one organisational culture view members of another in a stereotypical manner.

The case of community care

There were many instances of social work staff stating that all NHS personnel were dominated by 'the medical model', denying the social aspects of illness and dependency and favouring institutional care above community care. A senior social work manager said:

'I think we need to shift resources from the health service to community-based services rather than try to build up some kind of (health service) community resource and let the present level of medically orientated services continue',

and a senior social worker said:

'I feel that hospitals have a difficulty in getting people out into the community; partly it's what I call the mother hen syndrome - they're sometimes unwilling to take enough risks and maybe therefore they are not the best people to do that ... kind of thing. Or likewise perhaps they're overwilling to whip people back into hospital and it seems to be a constant dilemma'.

A basic grade social worker was sceptical of health service commitment to community care:

'Obviously I don't think they're putting their resources into the community. I mean if they were interested in doing that, they would. They haven't got enough commitment to it'.

And another basic grade social worker was of similar view:

'I think the hospital-type care is less good because of the medical model that is used in the hospitals and from my experience it does exclude the community'.

The picture presented from the social work side is of NHS personnel overwhelmingly opposed to the move towards community care - partly because of the dominance of 'the medical model', partly to protect the health service 'empire' and partly because of timidity (fear of taking risks). But when many of the health service responses are examined, it is clear that such a picture is a caricature of how health service personnel feel. A sector administrator, for example, said:

'I would say that if the patient can be cared for in the home and wants to stay home, that should be our ultimate aim although, you know, it may in the end cost more, and more people, social workers, home helps, people that are services, going in'.

And a senior nursing officer felt strongly about the need to preserve people's independence at home:

'I feel that no matter how humble a home, no matter how tatty it is, I think if an old person can hold on to a scrap of independence, I would certainly be all for trying very hard to help them keep that independence'.

Another senior nursing officer also had firm opinions:

'I would like to think it (community care) was people being maintained in their own homes ... I think it could still go much further ... If some of that money (spent on a residential unit) could have been channeled into the community, a good fifty per cent could have survived in the community ... and it would have been far better than spending all that and having them all in hospital'.

A district nurse saw community care as the policy for the future:

'I think it must be the nursing of the future ... with a much higher standard ... because now we're going in with this attitude that it's the total person and his family we're concerned with ... There's so much better care to give in the community if there's plenty of backup and support services, definitely'.

There were many other similar responses from health service personnel along these lines which brings into question the widely held view within social work that NHS staff tend to be opposed to the ideals of community care which social workers see themselves as holding. Such a division of perceptions was brought into play on a number of issues and this seems to support the proposition that allegiance to one's organisational group and its culture is in many ways as conditioning a factor as those of ideology and circumstance.

Conclusion

The very multiplicity of factors militating against the success of inter-professional working has consequences for attempts to improve collaboration. Whilst a commonality of experience sometimes confers similar attitudes and reactions on disparate groups of professionals, it frequently goes unrecognised; fundamental differences existing at the ideological level ensure that the gulf - and concomitant hostility - remains. This may then be exacerbated and, at times, superseded by ties of tribal allegiance which are not necessarily grounded in genuine differences of view but are, rather, the product of unfounded and stereotypical assumptions about those located outside the inclusive boundaries of organisation and culture. Attempts, therefore, to overcome ideological differences - through joint pre-qualifying or in-service training, for example - may fail because the strength of 'tribalism' goes unrecognised.

In current policy terms, this has interesting implications. At least two government-sponsored reports published in recent years have been concerned about divisions between the services involved in delivering health and social care at the community level. The Cumberlege report on community nursing,[18] for example, considered the establishment of a primary care authority in order to overcome some of the differences between community nurses (and their employing authorities, the district health authorities) and general practitioners (and their 'overseers', the family practitioner committees). The Griffiths report on community care,[19] on the other hand, recognised the fragmentation of community care services as they exist at present and advocated greater co-ordination by giving lead responsibility to social services departments. While both reports express admirable sentiments, it is unlikely that the recommendations of either could be entirely successful unless the complexity of inter-professional differences, and their causes, is fully recognised.

References

1. DHSS. Standing Medical Advisory Committee of the Central Health Services Council. *The Field of Work of the Family Doctor - Report of the Sub-Committee.* HMSO, London, 1963 (reprint) (The Dawson Report).

2. DHSS. Standing Medical Advisory Committee and Standing Nursing and Midwifery Advisory Committee. *The Primary Health Care Team.* HMSO, London, 1981 (The Harding Report).

3. DHSS. *Report of the Committee on Local Authority and Allied Personal Social Services.* Cmnd. 3703, HMSO, London, 1968 (The Seebohm Report)

4. DHSS. *Annual Report for 1974.* Cmnd. 6150, HMSO, 1975.

5. DHSS. *Priorities for Health and Personal Social Services in England - a Consultative Document.* HMSO, London, 1976.

6. DHSS. *Promoting Better Health - the Government's Programme for Improving Primary Health Care.* Cmnd. 249, HMSO, 1987 (The White Paper).

7. DHSS. *Report of the Inquiry into Child Abuse in Cleveland 1987.* Cm. 412, HMSO, London, 1988 (The Butler-Sloss Inquiry).

8. Strauss, A., Schatzman, L., Bucher, R., Erlich, D., and Sabshin, M. *Psychiatric Ideologies and Institutions.* Free Press of Glencoe and Collier Macmillan, London, 1964.

9. Marx, J.H. 'A Multidimensional Conception of Ideologies in Professional Arenas: the Case of the Mental Health Field' *Pacific Sociological Review*. 12, 2, 1969.

10. Mauksch, H.O. 'Ideology, Interaction and Patient Care in Hospitals' *Social Science and Medicine*. 7, 1973.

11. Smith, G. 'The Place of "Professional Ideology" in the Analysis of "Social Policy": Some Theoretical Conclusions from a Pilot Study of the Children's Panels' *Sociological Review*. 25, 1977.

12. Goldie, N. 'The Division of Labour Among the Mental Health Professions - a Negotiated or an Imposed Order'. In Stacey, M., Reid, M., Heath, C., and Dingwall, R. *Health and the Division of Labour*. Croom Helm, London, 1977.

13. Lonsdale, S., Webb, A., and Briggs, T.L. *Teamwork in the Personal Social Services and Health Care*. Croom Helm, London, 1980.

14. Bruce, N. *Teamwork for Preventive Care*. Research Studies Press, John Wiley and Sons Ltd., Chichester, 1981.

15. Dingwall, R. *The Social Organisation of Health Visiting Training*. Croom Helm, London, 1977.

16. Huntington, J. *Social Work and General Medical Practice: Collaboration or Conflict?* George Allen and Unwin, London, 1981.

17. Cartlidge, A., Bond, J., and Gregson, B. 'Interprofessional Collaboration in Primary Health Care' *Nursing Times*. 83, 46, 1987.

18. DHSS. *Neighbourhood Nursing - a Focus for Care*. HMSO, London, 1986 (The Cumberlege Report).

19. DHSS *Community Care: Agenda for Action*. HMSO, London, 1988

Groupwork in General Hospitals

Sheila Robertson

Introduction

This paper grew out of a professional involvement in some pieces of groupwork which were developed over the past ten years by social workers based in general hospitals in the Glasgow area. The involvement has been as an external consultant, and has seemed to come about in a rather haphazard (albeit enjoyable) way. The groupwork itself has also appeared to occur in a somewhat random fashion, with a sparse exchange of information or ideas between the hospitals, and little evidence that successful groupwork in one hospital has influenced developments elsewhere. Nonetheless, the cumulative effect has been suggestive of a growing interest in the use of groups, with an increasing willingness to include groupwork in a hospital social worker's repertoire of helping methods.

This seems an appropriate stage, then, at which to review groupwork developments within the Glasgow hospitals, and set these in a wider context. To do this, I have drawn on what is available in the literature and have also considered parallel work over a similar period of time in a hospital in Edinburgh. Pointers for policy and practice will emerge which may be helpful to social workers and their managers in health care settings.

The role of consultant

I must begin by clarifying my own role, since it verges on the idiosyncratic. For many years I have acted as external groupwork consultant to a range of projects in the West of Scotland, both in Strathclyde Social Work Department and in voluntary agencies. Within that consultancy work there has been a growing component of developments in general hospitals. In a typical example, a social worker and Senior might decide to set up a support group for patients recovering from a particular illness, to be run by the social worker and possibly a member of the medical staff. If they were uncertain about aspects of groupwork practice, and could not locate groupwork expertise among their colleagues, they might seek consultation outside. Advice at the planning stage, and help with practice issues which might emerge as the group progressed, would form the main focus for consultation; sometimes assistance in evaluating a group once it was over would also be requested. I would never, of course, attempt to take over the role of supervisor; accountability for service delivery has always (and properly) stayed with the Social Work Department.

The process of consultation has naturally varied, but there have been two common elements. The first has been the use of record material - and I have been impressed overall by the capacity of busy social workers to produce full and vivid accounts of group meetings. The second has been the regularity of discussions about the group (with social worker, with other staff who might be involved in the group, and possibly Senior Social Worker as well). My involvement might well be time limited (i.e. not for the total life of a group), but would certainly continue long enough, and be frequent enough, for me to develop a keen awareness of a group's viability and probable value to its members.

Sometimes there has been a very full role for the consultant; often, though, I have sensed that my usefulness has been as a provider of reassurance rather than as purveyor of otherwise unavailable groupwork lore. In other words, my function has been more as mascot and comforter, than as sage.

Sources

It must be clear from this description of role that I have amassed extremely detailed material about a particular set of groups, namely those in which I was involved as a consultant. Not surprisingly, it has been quite impractical to attempt to match this quantity and quality of data when considering wider areas of groupwork practice - even within the confines of the Glasgow hospital groups. All that I have been able to do in preparing this paper is acknowledge that I know a lot about a little, and try to work outwards from there.

First of all, I attempted to discover what else was going on in groupwork practice in general hospitals in Glasgow over the same time period. Sadly there seems to be a dearth of written material (articles, reports, evaluations, etc.); and changes in personnel have not helped: nonetheless I have managed to build up a general picture through discussion with hospital social work staff at many levels. I have also contacted social work managers at the Royal Infirmary in Edinburgh, in order to have 'matching' information about groupwork in a large hospital in another Scottish urban setting. To place this material in context, I have drawn on articles about specific examples of groupwork practice in general hospitals, using journals produced on both sides of the Atlantic. Finally, to provide an even broader framework, I have also considered how the use of groups in hospital social work 'fits' into general theoretical concepts about groupwork, and into perceptions of the role of social workers in health care.

A host of questions have burgeoned during this process of discussion and reading. How appropriate is the use of groups in a hospital social work setting? What prompts a social worker to start a group, and what sorts of support and supervision are necessary to provide a sound piece of practice? What do the consumers/members make of their group experiences? How do other hospital staff view groupwork? Why might there be a very successful group in one hospital, and no repeat elsewhere? How typical is the 'Glasgow experience'? What lessons can be drawn for subsequent practice? Should there be a policy initiative on the use of groups, or should developments be left to individual interest?

Many of these questions are alarming in their propensity for catching the investigator with too little data for a good answer. This paper tries to grapple with some of the issues raised, but can do no more than make a 'first offering'. What I have written is half-baked - or, at worst, the raw ingredients in the mixing bowl. Perhaps subsequent discussion among practitioners and managers will improve the balance of ingredients, and help the baking process on its way.

Groupwork theory and hospital social work

It seemed sensible to start with the broadest canvas, and address the basic question of the appropriateness of groupwork in a hospital setting. To do this some consideration of groupwork theory is unavoidable.

There are three main models of groupwork practice which enjoy a sizable following among social workers.[1] For the purposes of this paper I will focus on the 'mediating' or 'reciprocal' model expounded by Schwartz[2] and Shulman,[3] partly because I have used it as a theoretical underpinning for the consultancy work, and partly because it is by its very design especially appropriate for groupwork in institutional settings.

With the 'mediating' model, groupwork is seen as a way of helping a small group carry out its specific group tasks: this distinguishes the method from group therapy, which is less task oriented and is founded more in the medical pattern of diagnosis treatment - cure. In group therapy, the therapist uses the treatment of the individual members as the criterion for his intervention; in groupwork the worker intervenes principally when there is an obstacle to productive 'work'. (The work may be to create a mutual aid system to support parents of handicapped children; to carry out activities to develop social skills in long stay patients; to discuss and plan discharge from hospital to community ...).

The work of the group is established through an informal 'contract' between group members and agency, who agree upon this common area of tasks and purpose. Although this contract may need to be modified as time goes by and fresh needs emerge, it must be changed openly and honestly, as the members should all have an active stake in the work of the group. Clearly, the contractual perspective is valuable in establishing groups in institutional settings, by developing common ground between staff and residents or patients.[4]

In the opening chapter of his classic book *The Practice of Groupwork*, Schwartz describes what happened when a 'casework' agency began to provide a groupwork service to some of its clients.[2] He writes of the powerful effects of a helping process assisted by mutual aid, as people who have similar problems or shared similar life experiences came together to work on common tasks. The group members moved with 'amazing rapidity' into tackling the work; there seemed to be a release of anxiety flowing from the knowledge that difficult experiences or painful feelings were shared by all

Social workers and other professionals who undertake groupwork will recognise this phenomenon. In fact, there seems to be a kind of equation operating whereby the stronger the bond linking group members to each other and the clearer the factors that determine group membership, the more readily does the group move into serious work and the less likely are members to be distracted or deterred from the group task.

Clearly, these observations have relevance to groupwork in hospital settings. The 'centripetal' forces which draw group members to their agreed area of work are likely to be especially powerful when the shared experiences are of a serious, perhaps life threatening, illness ... and where people are all participating in a similar treatment regime in a ward. Patients in hospital are already 'grouped': even outpatients at a clinic, or relatives of patients, have an enormous amount in common. They are in crisis; differences in background, age, sex, race, may shade into insignificance compared with the crucial bond of illness, disfigurement, and worry and puzzlement over patterns of therapy. This is well described in an account of a discussion group held in the disorder of a waiting room of an oncology clinic:

> '... cohesiveness, mutual support, and discussion of common experiences emerged despite the informal, unstructured nature of the group. (It was) observed that the group members' experience of having cancer was the unifying factor that bound them together and outweighed all other considerations'.[5]

There are other reasons for supposing a hospital setting to be especially favourable for the use of groupwork. Not least is the 'captive' nature of the population of prospective group members (which is certainly not the same as saying that all patients are eager or compliant group members - they rightly retain a genuine capacity for opting out). Establishing who is eligible to join a group, and enabling them to attend, is obviously a far less fraught process in hospital than in the community, and should in theory give groupwork initiatives a secure and encouraging start.

Both general and psychiatric hospitals have long traditions of the use of group methods by disciplines other than social work. Occupational therapists have a particularly substantial record of work with groups - as have psychiatrists, psychologists and nurses in psychiatric hospitals with a 'therapeutic community' style of treatment. How much this might influence social workers contemplating groupwork in general hospitals is hard to say: it would seem to be a helpful precedent and should provide opportunities for collaboration in the use of group methods.

There is a further point to consider - namely, the institutionalising effect upon patients of a prolonged stay in even the most sympathetically run of hospital wards. Counteracting this effect is far from easy, but the provision of group meetings to air collective discontent with the ward regime, and to open up communications among patients, and between patients and staff, may be helpful.[6] This suggests that a hospital is a setting which not only favours the development of groups where the focus is on individual worries and individual rehabilitation, but also demands serious consideration of groupwork to mitigate the effects of institutionalisation.

This adds up to an impressive and persuasive argument for the use of groupwork - an argument which flows from a number of practice-based considerations. We might therefore expect every social worker located in a hospital to be a groupworker as well as an individual and family counsellor ... and groups involving social workers and other medical staff to be active in nooks and crannies in most parts of a general hospital.

Yet, of course, this is not so. Not only from my own observations in Glasgow, but from studying the literature and from discussion with hospital social workers in other areas, it is clear that groupwork is still a relatively uncommon way of delivering a service in health care social work. Indeed, this is true in other branches of social work also (except perhaps services to children).[7]

Clearly, there must be countervailing forces at work. The first which springs to mind is the continuing low profile given to groupwork on many social work training courses. Even where a reasonable theoretical input may exist, there is a regrettable tendency to provide placement experiences which are observational, or, at best, allow a student to be a 'back up' to another social worker in a pre-established group. Very few students, once qualified, feel confident to go solo as groupworkers; and here there is a striking contrast with the United States, where groupwork has been long established as a viable social work method, and hospitals have long been regarded as a suitable venue for its practice.[8]

I think the other countervailing forces arise from what are basically organisational issues. For social workers, enthusiasm for attempting a time consuming and innovatory piece of work will obviously be dampened by the effects of staff shortages, changeover in personnel, and restructuring - and many Social Work Departments have experienced all or some of these problems recently. Within the hospital structure itself, further built-in difficulties exist. Firstly, there is the need to communicate fully and rapidly with consultants, nurses, and other medical staff when a group is being developed. Once this is done, the group becomes a very public concept ... and if it 'fails', the unfortunate instigator will not be able to avoid comment and criticism. It requires a very committed social worker to contemplate such a visible test of skill. Moreover, the nature of a hospital as a provider of health care means that the medical model permeates the very brickwork: professional opinions and decisions dominate; patients acquiesce. Gathering patients in groups, and implicitly or explicitly giving them licence to query or criticise their treatment, may antagonise medical staff and upset social worker-doctor relationships unless this whole process is handled sensitively.

The Glasgow experience

From a practice perspective, then, groupwork seems a highly appropriate way of providing a social work service in hospital. From an organisational perspective, however, it is a far less inviting prospect. How has this balance of opposing influences worked out in the Glasgow hospitals?

Strathclyde Region Social Work Department is divided into twelve Districts, four of which cover Glasgow. My own consultancy work has been limited to six of the non-psychiatric hospitals, spread across three of the Districts. I have contacted social work staff and management with particular responsibility for health care in all four Districts, to widen the picture to include any groupwork undertaken in recent years. Changes in personnel mean that some of the groupwork can only be dated approximately, and I cannot be sure of having covered all groupwork developments. However, the overall picture is appreciably less sketchy than if I had limited consideration to my own consultancy work.

The groupwork undertaken in Glasgow can be divided into three main categories: for patients suffering from specific illnesses or disabilities; for relatives of such patients; and for elderly residents in long stay wards. It has been possible to find examples from the literature and from groupwork practice in the Royal Infirmary in Edinburgh (my other source of comparisons) which 'match' the work in all three categories. In a sense, I regard this matching as a sort of crude validation process confirming the Glasgow experience as falling well within the mainstream of groupwork developments in hospitals. By establishing the work in Glasgow as 'typical', the pointers for practice and ideas for future development which have emerged from that area may with confidence be considered to have a wider application. This is not at all a rigorous way of going about things, but is probably rather better than turning the spotlight on Glasgow and failing to make useful connections with practice elsewhere.

It would have been interesting to go further, and establish whether there have been significant variations between the amount of groupwork undertaken in different hospitals, and in different areas of Scotland. If variations have emerged, then an intriguing search for explanations could follow. Unfortunately, this has been well beyond the scope of my enquiry, and would anyway have been especially hard to achieve in places where the turnover of social work personnel has been high.

The Glasgow experience: groupwork categories

In addition to the three main categories mentioned above there are two others which need to be discussed briefly here before being set aside. The first involves setting up branches or local groupings to link with national organisations such as Tac Tent, Headway and the Parkinson's Disease Association. Many of the Glasgow hospitals have such affiliated groups, often with consultants as the main instigators, and with social workers as part of a staff component of membership. These are important groups, but by definition are outwith the main thrust of this paper, which is towards work with small groups initiated by social workers in response to identified needs arising out of their workload. The second category involves work with groups which have an essentially recreational remit - for example, a sports club for paraplegic patients, or an entertainment club for frail elderly residents. While not wishing to detract from the importance of these groups to the participants, it is not clear that setting up and working with such a group is a specific social work function.

The three principal categories remain: groups for patients with particular illnesses or disabilities; groups for relatives of such patients; and groups for elderly patients on long stay wards. Each of these categories is discussed separately below, with examples given from Glasgow hospitals and from articles in social work or medical journals.

(i) Groups for patients with a specific diagnosis

Examples of these from the Glasgow area include a group for amputees,[9] a group for head injured patients and their relatives, and a group for women suffering from pre-menstrual tension. The first two are 'rolling' groups with a slowly changing membership; the last has been short term. Equivalent instances from the literature include groups for heart patients,[10] cancer patients,[5] and amputees.[11]

The main characteristic of all these groups is the focus on the diagnosis or condition. Much of the group's work is around giving and receiving information about the illness, about treatment and prognosis, and about ways of coping. Anxieties are shared, and support given not only by the groupworker but by members to each other. Such groups tend to meet within hospital walls; and may include medical staff as well as social workers among the professionals who attend. The main purpose is clearly to aid rehabilitation, and all groups emphasise the value of expressing feelings, gaining understanding, and providing mutual encouragement when the going is rough.

(ii) Groups for relatives of patients

Glasgow examples include groups for relatives of stroke victims, and for parents of children who have had severe burns. In the literature there are matching examples of groups for parents of children with Cystic Fibrosis;[12] groups for spouses of renal patients;[13] groups for patients mourning the loss of a child from cancer;[14] and support groups for relatives of dementia patients.[15,16]

These groups meet for varying time durations and sometimes in venues outside hospitals. Sometimes there is a low takeup rate for membership, and there may be difficulties in integrating members who have adjusted in very varying ways to their relative's illness, deterioration or even death. In other words, these groups show much more fragmentation than those in the preceding category; presumably this is because the focus for discussion - the ill relative - is at one remove from the group members themselves, and for practical reasons attendance may be difficult.

(iii) Groups for elderly long stay patients

In Glasgow there have been a series of such groups for frail ambulant residents in one hospital, and short term groups in geriatric wards in another. The literature includes a description of similar work in a small group for elderly people,[17] and parallel experiences in groupwork in old people's homes.[4]

The focus of all these groups is on providing a stimulating meeting, with the aim of improving communication among patients, and also providing some opportunity for them to influence their environment by discussing complaints, suggestions for entertainments, etc. with care staff. Discussion may range widely from events which took place sixty years ago to those which occurred yesterday! The groupworkers try to make sure that everyone has an opportunity to speak, and may make imaginative use of pictures, slides, or other devices to encourage discussion and rouse people's imaginations and memories.

The Glasgow experience: some questions discussed and lessons learned

At the start of this paper I identified a number of questions which arose naturally from reading, discussion and a general review of groupwork practice in Glasgow hospitals. Two of these questions have now been tackled: viz, the appropriateness of groupwork as a helping method in hospital social work, and the extent to which the Glasgow Experience may be regarded as 'typical', at least in terms of the kinds of groups set up and the programmes of work undertaken by group members. Further questions remain to be considered.

(i) What prompts a social worker to set up a particular group?

As one social worker commented to me, the need for a specific group 'hits you in the face'. A ground swell of grumbles in a ward; a cluster of families receiving counselling for similar problems and worries; patients at a clinic getting together informally to offer each other support ... these are the sorts of events which will prompt consideration of a groupwork service. For a social worker to be responsive to such prompting, additional factors need to prevail. I have found that workers who take up the groupwork challenge usually have the following characteristics: they are very experienced in hospital social work (and consequently well equipped to negotiate the organisational aspects of setting up a group); they are especially experienced in providing counselling in relation to the illness or disability for which groupwork is being contemplated (it may even be termed their 'specialism'); their workload may be heavy, but will not be cripplingly so; and their supervisor is prepared to encourage and enthuse. Sometimes other hospital staff are keen to act as co-workers in the proposed group, and this additional injection of support and encouragement is often a helpful spur to action.

Interestingly, I have not encountered social workers who were rabid devotees of groupwork as a method! This is probably because well established hospital social work staff will have qualified some time ago, when groupwork was very unlikely to have formed a significant part of their training. The impetus has come more from a professional confidence and competence, combined with the recognition that individual and family counselling cannot adequately help in certain situations which might be more responsive to some form of group approach.

(ii) What sorts of supervision or consultation are desirable?

In an ideal world, supervision would be able to provide as full a range of support and advice for groupwork as for the more traditional forms of hospital social work. At the moment this is not always possible, and social workers and supervisors risk floundering at the crucial planning stage, when group composition and initial contracts with prospective members are important and vexed issues which need a confident resolution. Some form of additional support through consultation may be necessary. The Royal Infirmary in Edinburgh used a senior member of its social work team to provide such consultation; my own role in Glasgow has probably been less effective, because of my separation from the Social Work Department, but nonetheless has been helpful in getting a number of competent pieces of groupwork practice off the ground. Clearly, some variation on the thought of internal consultation provided in Edinburgh or external consultation provided by myself in Glasgow would seem desirable.

(iii) What do the consumers/clients make of their group experiences?

The expressed enthusiasm of group members for the service that has been provided for them has been striking. One might expect this to be true of the groups which have been written up (no one is likely to record a disaster), but I found it to be true also of all the groups of which I have close knowledge. The enthusiasm was not just for an opportunity to meet other patients or relatives and enjoy a break from the usual hospital routine: group members were able and willing to identify further benefits the giving and receiving of support and information, a relief from anxiety, and the learning of more appropriate ways of coping with a difficult situation. For many group members there was also the opportunity to see social workers and medical staff in a new and more informal light, which subsequently enabled them to make better use of their professional services.

(iv) What lessons can be drawn for subsequent practice?

I have been very struck by two aspects of the groupwork practice that I have encountered in my consultancy work. The first relates to the transferability of skills from individual counselling to work in groups. Social workers who were extremely doubtful of their ability to cope with the 'mysteries' of groupwork quickly realised that the fundamentals of social work with one person, two, or many are the same. The use of self, use of time, clarity in carrying out of agency function, and an adherence to the need for a contract openly and honestly arrived at - these are as important and valuable in groupwork as in individual counselling. Setting up a group, and dealing with the complexities of group composition, may seem to be overwhelmingly strange and puzzling at first; but with some advice, and logical application of the fundamentals of social work practice, they need not be daunting to an experienced practitioner.[3]

The second aspect is less to do with direct work with clients and more with negotiating the hospital environment. The most frequently occurring difficulty encountered by social workers (despite all their care) arose when group members in some way fell foul of medical staff: by being temporarily unavailable for treatment, taking up room space for a meeting that was needed by someone else, or by questioning their treatment. At times the very survival of a group might be threatened, as medical wrath descended upon it. However accustomed social workers may be to working in a secondary setting like a hospital, they need to continue to invest as much skill and sensitivity in contacts with the staff as in contacts with clients.

I have one final comment in relation to groupwork practice. As I have already indicated, there seems to be in the Glasgow area a lack of written material about the groupwork that has been undertaken in the past. I am not referring to the keeping of records - rather the writing up of a group once it has been finished, with some conclusion about its value, and some indications of how subsequent work in a similar vein might best be tackled. Sometimes social workers attempting groupwork must have felt that they were recreating the wheel; whereas a 'bank' of information about groupwork already undertaken of a similar nature would have helped them avoid repeating mistakes, and would have given them encouragement for the ultimate success of their enterprise.

The Edinburgh experience

Over the last decade the Royal Infirmary in Edinburgh has enjoyed the favourable circumstances of retaining a number of senior and extremely experienced social work staff, and this situation has been highly propitious for the practice of group-work (as my earlier comments might suggest). One of the social work staff described the Department as 'bubbling' with ideas and enthusiasm; certainly it seems that there were a number of staff who proved able to carry out groupwork to a high level of skill. The renal and heart surgery units in particular have been settings for exten-sive groupwork practice over virtually the entire time period under consideration. I found when I consulted staff at the Infirmary that the collective 'memory' of the groups that had been developed was very good - and quite a lot of writing up had been done, so it would seem unlikely that this experience will ever be 'lost' in the future. The presence of an internal supporter/consultant for groupwork probably contributed not only to success in the use of group methods, but also to the devel-opment of this 'memory bank'.

Conclusions

I think the conclusions to this paper should really form the answer to the final ques-tion as to whether the development of groups should be a matter of policy or left to individual enterprise. I have come to feel increasingly strongly that there would be a value in social work managers in health care actively encouraging the development of groupwork in all appropriate hospital settings. To continue with the individual in-itiative approach will not enable a coherent and consistent level of practice to be es-tablished - and there is a clear need for some central organising of information about groups that have been developed, about lessons learnt, and about the circumstan-ces under which groups are most likely to flourish. The identification of people with-in the Social Work Department who can act as consultants may be a useful additional source of support and skill enhancement. The ultimate benefits to clients seem to be beyond question.

References

1. Papell, C., and Rothman, B. 'Social Groupwork Models: Possession and Heritage' *Journal of Education for Social Work.* 2, 2, 1966, 66-77.

2. Schwartz, W., and Zalba, S. (eds.) *The Practice of Groupwork.* Columbia University Press, New York, 1971.

3. Shulman, L. *The Skills of Helping Individuals and Groups.* Peacock, Illinois, 1984.

4. Sturton, S. 'Developing Groupwork in a Casework Agency' *British Journal of Social Work.* 2, Summer 1972, 144-158.

5. Arnowitz, E., Brunswick, L., and Kaplan, B. 'Group Therapy for Oncology Patients' *Social Work*. 28, 5, September-October 1983, 397.

6. Weiner, H. 'The Hospital, the Ward and the Patient as Clients: Use of the Group Method' *Social Work*. 4, 4, October 1959, 57-64.

7. Preston-Shoot, M. 'Groupwork, Challenges and Rewards' *Social Work Today*. 18, 27, March 1987.

8. Frey, L. (ed.) *Use of Groups in the Health Field*. National Association of Social Workers, New York, 1966.

9. Cottey, P., Robertson, S., Scott, H., and Thompson, R. 'The Amputees' Group: An Interim Evaluation'. Paper presented at I.S.P.O. Conference, Bath, 1988.

10. Clarke, J., and McBean, I. 'Group Therapy with Heart Attack Patients' *Social Work Today*. 10, I, August 1978, 17-18.

11. Lipp, M., and Malone, S. 'Group Rehabilitation of Vascular Surgery Patients' *Archive of Physical Medical Rehabilitation*. 57, April 1976, 180-183.

12. Bywater, M. 'Coping with a Life-Threatening Illness: An Experiment in Parents' Groups' *British Journal of Social Work*. 14, 1984, 117-127.

13. Held over the past ten years at the Renal Unit in the Royal Infirmary, Edinburgh.

14. Otech, C., and Soricelli, B. 'Mourning the Death of a Child' *Social Work*. 30, 5, September-October 1985.

15. Fuller, J., Ward, E., Massam, K., and Gardner, A. 'Dementia: Supportive Groups for Relatives' *British Medical Journal*. 1, 1979, 1684-1685.

16. Cantley, C., and Smith, G. 'Social Work and a Relatives' Support Group in a Psychogeriatric Day Hospital: A Research Note' *British Journal of Social Work*. 13, 1983, 663-670.

17. Hunter, J. 'A Shared Reality for Old People' *Social Work Today*. 13, 10, November 1981.

Health Centre Social Work - Plugging the Gap?
A Comparative Study of Client Groups Using
a Health Centre and an Area Office

D. A. Cairns Smith

Introduction

This paper has modest origins and ambitions. I was a new appointment, the first social worker in a Health Centre which had itself only opened two years previously. It seemed sensible to monitor what was happening and use the information as a basis for evaluation and planning at the end of my first year. Like other contributors I firmly believe that if social workers want to improve their practice, some evaluation, albeit subjective, is essential. My study involved the use of a referral analysis 'tick sheet' prepared by Strathclyde Region to monitor client groups using Area Office social services. The personal circumstances of the client, the referral process, the problems, and the services provided were logged and then compared with the statistics gathered in the local Area Office over the same period in order to see whether there were any significant differences. The findings are compared with previous studies by other researchers in health-based settings and in some instances examples are given of specific work with clients.

The setting

Barrhead is a small industrial town on the outskirts of Glasgow, with a population of about 35,000. Because of a decline in manufacturing industry in the area, unemployment is a major problem running at about twenty-five per cent with a much higher ratio (circa seventy-five per cent) in certain housing estates. One of these has been designated as an 'Area of Priority Treatment' (APT), by Strathclyde Region. There is a high input of social work in this estate. Two villages are also included in the catchment area of both surveys.

The population is a mixture of native families, who have lived in the area for generations, and 'in-comers', mainly Glasgow 'overspill' families, who moved into the newly built council estates. This seems to have changed the character of the town, eroding much of the community spirit which was evident seventeen years ago when I first worked in the area. There seems to be, for example, more theft than there used to be.

The Health Centre in 1982 covered 22,000 patients in four, later five, practices. The social worker was technically attached to the largest practice consisting of five doctors. However, the location of her room in the midst of the four small practices meant that all sought advice, often of a quick information-seeking nature. ('Where can I send Mrs X to get a benefit check?' Answer; 'Wheel her in and I'll see her.') If the client was seen briefly, these contacts were not logged as a referral. This made for very easy and informal contact between the social worker and the medical profession and this in turn often saved a client a half mile journey up a steepish hill to the area office. The location of the Centre, opposite the main shopping precinct with the Post Office immediately across the road, also made it a well-used community resource.

Method

Choosing a method of evaluation was easy. The Area Office in which I had worked before coming to the Health Centre had been involved in a pilot study using the Referral Analysis 'tick sheet' prepared by the research department of Strathclyde Region (Appendix A). The Area Office in Barrhead had recently adopted these 'tick sheets' to look at its practice. To extend this to the Health Centre seemed logical and enabled me to make a direct comparison with the Area Office findings.

Taking the seven months from October 1982 to April 1983 inclusive, the Area Office survey covered 474 clients and the Health Centre sixty-one. I continued the survey in the Centre to cover the same seven months in 1983-4 when seventy-nine clients were seen. It is perhaps worth mentioning that there tends to be a hidden caseload, especially in the Health Centre, of people who 'catch you in passing'. A number of ex-clients seem to lie in wait, perhaps seeking advice about a financial problem or about a relative or friend or about what to say to the doctor. These do not appear in the analysis. Another excluded category are those who 'pop in' to let one know the outcome of advice given and then ask about other problems that are concerning them. In addition, members of staff often sought help with personal problems on an informal oasis. This included cleaners, consultants, receptionists and para-medical staff.

Analysis of results

1. Referral Process

The 'tick-sheets' contained a post code which enabled one to delineate areas of high demand and a dating system (see Appendix A). There was no significant seasonal variation. Clients were mainly from estates owned by the District Council, and indeed, from a relatively small number of streets within the estates, but no area was exempt. Both settings showed similar patterns. There were significant differences in the two settings in the methods of referral and the referrer.

Figure 1. Method of Referral

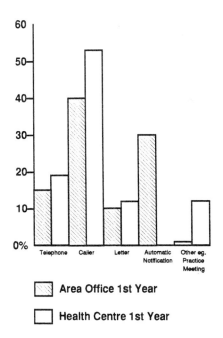

The chart shows that the Area Office received twenty-eight per cent of its referrals as 'automatic notifications'. These consist of requests from the court, or the Reporter to the Children's Hearing, for social background reports. These reports are always allocated to social workers to investigate and complete. There are also notifications from the housing departments or fuel boards indicating eviction or disconnection proceedings. In these cases a letter is usually sent offering an appointment. While I was given a share of these reports as part of my workload they do not appear in the Health Centre statistics.

GPs sometimes referred their patient by letter in order to log the referral in their case records. They would also telephone me if the patient was in the surgery and they wanted them seen quickly. The usual method of referral was by personal contact at practice meetings or by calling in to my room. This enabled them to give me a much fuller picture of the patient's problem and background history. Michael Sheppard[1] in his research into the reaction of GPs to social workers stated that

> 'the quality and frequency of communication varied according to the type of problem, perceived attitude of the GP and occupation of the worker.'

This was certainly my experience. In other cases, such as financial advice, GPs tended to suggest that their patient make an appointment to see me. These were logged as 'callers' on the chart. Many of these callers revealed further problems once their initial worries were dealt with.

It had been decided, prior to my appointment, by senior managers in the social work and health departments that all Health Centre referrals would come from the largest GP practice. However, other GPs, health visitors, district nurses and occasionally consultants also referred patients. While this was discouraged by my department, since it ignored the official social work channels, it was not resented by the 'big practice' since I was used mainly in a short-term, advisory capacity. The 'self' referrals were from people that the GPs or receptionists had steered in my direction. This also applied to relatives who were often seeking respite care for elderly or disabled relations and who also badly needed to discuss their feelings about the difficulties of being a 'carer', however willing. In my second year many clients referred themselves or friends to me, again by-passing the official system.

The low referral rate by GPs to the Area team was also noted in Sheppard's research[1] which showed that in spite of 'the broad and positive stated interpretation by GPs of the Social Work role' they only referred an average of four to eight patients per year and this was mainly for practical or resource help.

Figure 2. Referrer

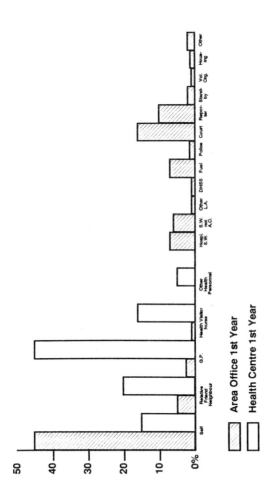

Figure 3. Sex Referral Status

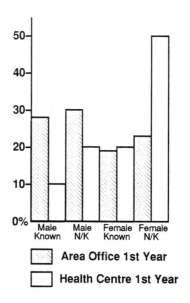

2. The Client

Details of the client's sex, marital status, age, living group and financial circumstances were recorded.

From Figure 3 it can be seen that seventy per cent of Health Centre referrals were women compared with about forty per cent in the Area Office. Over seventy per cent of Health Centre clients had never seen a social worker before and those that had contacted the department had seen either the occupational therapist or home-help organiser. In almost every case the clients prefaced their remarks by assuring me that they would not have 'gone to the Welfare' and had only come to see me to please the Doctor. The notion of 'stigma' was clearly felt and somehow the Health Centre escaped this. M.E. Jenkin's work on the attachment of social workers

Figure 4. Age Band

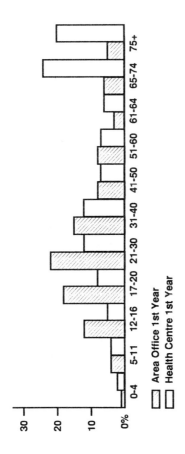

to GP practices[2] made a similar observation; the GPs themselves indicated a preference for patients to be seen in surgeries because they felt it was a more acceptable setting. This was also borne out by June Huntington's research.[3] In her unpublished report[4] she suggested that patients saw the social worker in the Health Centre 'as an extension of the doctor'. The Health Centre as a source of new client groups is referred to in a number of studies, notably in the work of Roslyn Corney.[5] Her findings also reflect the age band and living group differences in the two settings.

The age band chart (figure 4) shows clearly that Area Office clients tend to be younger, perhaps because of the large demand for social background reports for Hearings and the Court in this age group. In the Health Centre, however, I saw a number of women in the age group twenty to forty who were experiencing relationship difficulties. I also found that forty per cent of my clients were over sixty-five, most of them living alone.

Figure 5 shows that many pensioners living alone used the service in the Health Centre. The location almost certainly contributed to this. They visited the Centre for chiropody as well as medical treatment; the Area Office, although only half a mile away, involved a walk uphill. The reason given by clients was again reluctance to seek social work help. Most had a fear of 'not managing'. They 'did not want to ask for "charity"'. It often took all my powers of persuasion to get them to apply for the additional grants to which they were entitled. I can only think of one case in the five years I worked in the Centre where an elderly client was on the correct benefit; most under-claimed by between £2 and £5 per week. I can think of several who, when advised of their entitlement, refused to approach DHSS whom they often confused with the Social Work Department. Stigma again seemed to be the main deterrent.

Forty-four per cent of Health Centre referrals were from people who had been widowed or whose marriages had broken down. Many expressed loneliness and they often found themselves discussing their loss, still very painful even after many years. Few had originally come to talk about this aspect of their life, or would have seen themselves as in need of bereavement counselling. Many returned to tell me the result of their claims and they frequently used the opportunity to talk again about their sadness.

In the Health Centre retirement benefit accounted for thirty-three per cent of referrals compared with eight per cent in the Area Office. The other categories are similar though usually slightly higher in the Area Office. 'Not applicable' applies to children referred. I had expected that more clients might be working. Corney and Bowen's research[6] indicated that

'Intake clients were more likely to be unemployed, living on benefits, in council or rented accommodation ... The attachment group on the other hand, had more

Figure 5. Living Group

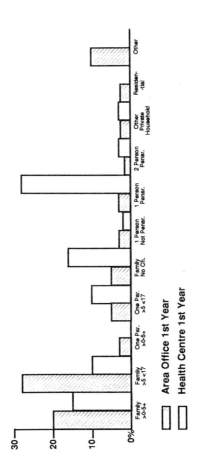

Figure 6. Marital Status

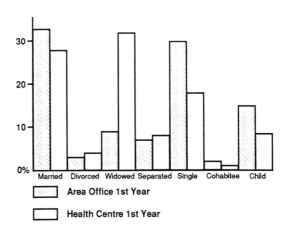

women referred who were either housewives or working, living on their own earnings or their husbands. Their clients were more likely to own their own homes.'

My findings did not show this but the difference might be explained by the differences in location between the studies. In my second year in the Centre I continued to complete 'tick sheets' but I did not include clients in receipt of sickness or invalidity benefit in the supplementary benefit category, as I had done in my first year. This increased the percentage on sickness or invalidity benefit from five per cent to nineteen per cent, reducing supplementary benefit claimants by half.

These findings were more in tune with those of Goldberg and Neill[7] who showed in their study, carried out in the early 1970s, that people of all social classes used the health based service.

Figure 7. Benefit

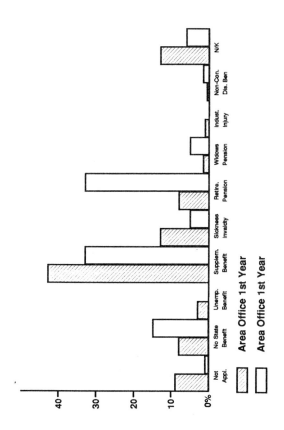

Figure 8. Primary Reasons for Referral

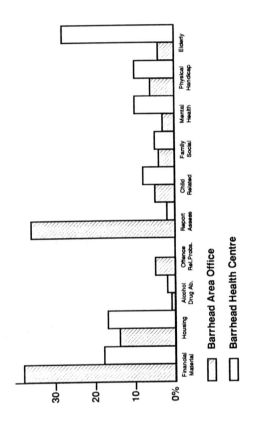

3. Reasons for referral

About half of the Area Office referrals were to do with financial or housing problems as was the case with nearly twenty per cent of Health Centre referrals. These were mainly dealt with on a one-off, no further action basis. In a comprehensive study of referral, unfortunately never published, McLaren and McLean produced similar results overall.[8] In the Paisley study however 23.2 per cent of Area Office clients were elderly, a difference which may be partly explained by the 'patch-based' input by health visitors in Barrhead and by the fact that the pensioners in the area often have relatives living locally or have themselves lived for many years in the same house and have support from neighbours. Many health-based referrals were for respite care, benefit advice or because of increasing mental or physical frailty.

In the Area Office less than thirty per cent of 'tick-sheets' had secondary reasons logged. When tertiary reasons were logged only eight per cent of sheets were ticked. These were evenly divided between financial, housing, child care, mental and physical problems. This was similar in the Paisley Area Office study[8] where 72.5 per cent had no secondary and 92.5 per cent no tertiary problem identified. In the Health Centre only a quarter of clients had no secondary, and a half no tertiary problem identified. The figures collated in my second year study showed 8 per cent with no obvious secondary reasons and twenty-five per cent with no obvious tertiary reasons for referral.

There seem to me to be several possible reasons for these differences between the two settings. Firstly, there was perhaps less commitment to completing the forms accurately in the Area Office. Secondly, all reports were logged by administrative staff who may not have known the clients and might therefore have been unable to pick out other problems. A third reason may lie in the physical setting itself. Area Office waiting rooms can be somewhat off-putting. They are often bedecked with posters reinforcing the problems or inadequacies of the client. There are often no toys for the children. There may well be a queue of people waiting. Many interview rooms lack telephones. In the Health Centre the room was cosy with comfortable chairs, toys, books and posters from art galleries on the walls. There was a telephone which meant that clients could not only hear what was being said about them but also, in the endless delays being shunted around the various sections of DHSS for example, problems could be explored further.

Another important factor is in the amount of information available at the start of the interview. I believe this accounts for the difference in numbers of secondary and tertiary reasons identified during my first and second year in the Health Centre. As the GPs learned to trust me and I was able to demonstrate some skills in counselling, in addition to wielding a calculator for a benefit check, the referrals tended

Figure 9. Secondary Reason for Referral

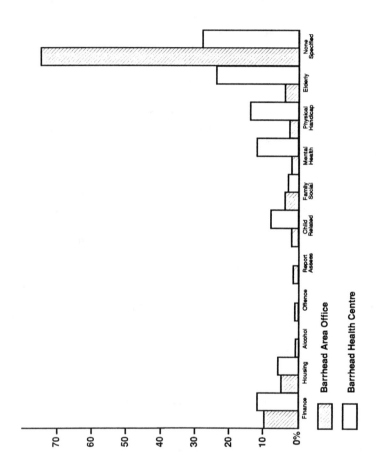

to be more detailed, more helpful and indeed more appropriate. It was then easier to steer discussion into more sensitive areas. It was also a more direct discussion. Patients are used to having a very limited time with their GPs and so have to come straight to the point often on very personal matters. They somehow seemed to treat the social worker in much the same way.

One example of this was a young woman whom the Health Visitor had referred to me. She appeared at my door clutching a baby and saying 'Doctor's sent me doon aboot the sex. I cannae abide it and she says you'll sort it oot!'. One cannot be more direct than that. Having checked with the client and the GP that the problem was more to do with ignorance and poor technique than any deep rooted psychological hang-up I was able to work on a weekly basis with her and her husband. We consulted the GP as appropriate. At the end of three to four months the problems were largely resolved. My 'proof' of this lies in the clients themselves who informed me that their neighbours were also experiencing sexual problems and 'So we tellt them jist tae see you'.

Another major factor is time. In a busy Area Office there is a temptation to deal only with the presenting problem, offering a second appointment if further problems are suspected. An example of this is an elderly man who frequented the office with various financial worries. When investigating these issues it was clear he was very well informed about benefit regulations. It was only on probing further that it emerged that his wife had died 18 months before. He was lonely and depressed and used the office as a point of social contact. Referral to local lunch clubs, not DHSS, was what he needed.

While many of the presenting problems in both settings were of a practical nature there were often, in the Health Centre at least, underlying stresses to do with isolation, coming to terms with illness or handicap in oneself or a relative, or strained personal relationships. By focussing on these early, before the unforgivable has been said or done, or before the strain of caring has become too trying, a client was often able to break the problem into manageable bits or let off steam sufficiently to keep coping.

Clients coming to an Area Office for help with these personal crises are often at a stage beyond this. Winny and Corney[9] referred to the many studies which reflect on the preventative nature of health based work

> 'especially with marital, emotional and family problems. Clients are referred at an earlier stage, for example when marital or child care difficulties are just beginning, rather than when these are severe, chronic and less easy to change.'

This seems to them to provide a sound economic argument for extending health based social work.

Figure 10. Allocation

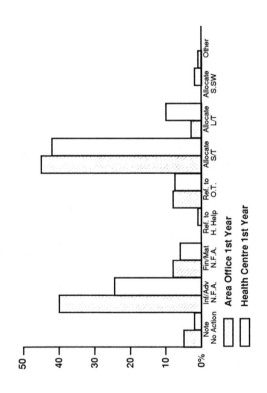

Goldberg and Neill[7] found that people from different social classes presented different problems.

'Family problems, many of them revealing very disturbed relationships, were more often presented by clients from the professional and managerial classes, while problems related to ill health, both physical and mental, were more concentrated among patients in semi and unskilled occupations.'

It was certainly true that the professional and managerial families who consulted me were often having relationship problems either with teenage children or elderly relatives. Some consulted me about marital problems where sexual frustration or alcohol abuse were also factors. These problems were however equally common in other socio-economic classes. I often found that a one-off lesson in communication using, for example, Transactional Analysis in the style of Berne,[10] was a valuable tool in helping families see where problems were arising.

4. Allocation patterns

More than half Area Office referrals were not allocated or were passed on to the occupational therapist. Of the remainder almost thirty per cent were requests for reports which were automatically allocated. In the Health Centre 42.6 per cent of referrals were allocated for short term involvement and nearly ten per cent for long term support. The latter tended to be cases of chronic illness, both mental and physical. In one case a boy of seven was found to be suffering from a severe, progressive debilitating illness. In less than two years he went from being a slightly clumsy boy, attending the local primary school, to being without speech, unable to move and finally tube-fed. Helping his parents, his brother and in the early stages the boy himself, come to terms with this involved a multidiscipline team consisting of two consultants, GP, speech therapist, health visitor, social worker, occupational therapist and respite care staff as well as educational staff. Being largely under one roof was a major factor in facilitating communication. It is almost certain that this case would not have been referred to the area team and indeed was 'closed' when I left the Health Centre. My task had been one of mobilising resources from statutory and voluntary agencies but also involved hours of patient listening.

A primary care team as such did not exist but was an *ad hoc* arrangement dictated by the nature of each individual case. Terminal care is an obvious example, again not likely to be referred by the GP to social workers until he has got to know their skills, but where a social worker may be able to offer an added dimension. Winny and Rushton[11] quote a GP who stated that she no longer reached for her prescription pad when seeing a distressed patient, knowing she can refer to a social worker. They also point out that

'When the social worker visits a client it sometimes emerges that the client was afraid to contradict the doctor's advice.'

The GP may well have misunderstood the client's feelings. The following case I dealt with is an example. A forty-year-old woman was diagnosed as having cancer. She had already had two mastectomies and was experiencing pain under the scarring and in her lymph glands and chest. The GP, into whose area she had just moved, tried to reassure her about her illness and sent me to sort out financial and marital problems. What she shared with me was her great anxiety that the doctor was not taking her condition seriously and was unaware of how ill she was. When this was passed on to the GP he was able to change his tack and be much more direct. I was then able to help her contact and arrange visits from relatives, obtain financial help and contact her estranged husband who returned to support the family through the last months. The health visitor and specialist nurses from the Macmillan Fund provided medical support. She was a brave and dignified woman who took great comfort in having reconciled her husband and children before she died.

5. Option boxes

There were four option boxes provided to enable more flexible use to be made of the analysis forms. One was used to obtain information for the Region about social work clients who had been employed by Chrysler (their Linwood factory had recently closed) to see whether this had created demands on social services. This did not seem to be a major factor in Barrhead. I used the second box to identify the type of help I was seeking from the Occupational Therapy section. The third box was used to identify the medical referrer by name. This showed that the more experienced GPs made most use of my services. Younger GPs referred financial or housing problems but preferred to do their own bereavement or terminal counselling. Clients often appreciated the doctor's concern but felt they had not liked to impose on a busy GP's time and that when they really needed help, often months after the death, the GP had ceased to call. As I became better known the ratio changed slightly. The final box specified the nature of the illness suffered by the referred patient. About twenty-five per cent had mental illnesses, ranging from anxiety to psychosis, and a further twenty-five per cent illnesses to do with the heart or lungs. The remaining fifty per cent included patients with a variety of conditions including multiple sclerosis, cancer, pregnancy and paralysis.

Conclusion

There was nothing startlingly new about my findings in the Health Centre. There have been a number of studies, some of which I have referred to in the text, which my data largely reinforces. What was interesting was the opportunity to make a direct comparison with an area team covering the same catchment area and using the same data base over the same period of time. This showed clearly that the local team missed out on certain groups of clients, many of whom were elderly, ill and isolated. They presented with a variety of problems, often multiple, and came from all walks of life. Many were explicit that they would not have used the Area Office service because of the stigma which they felt was attached to the Social Work Department. It also showed that GPs were not prepared to refer sensitive issues such as bereavement counselling to the team. This observation has also been made previously,

> 'Before we moved into the Health Centre we didn't use social workers to anything like the same extent ... Doctors who decry social workers have never worked with them'.[12]

The allocation pattern indicated that many of the cases allocated in the Health Centre would not have been allocated in the area team, if indeed the extent of the problem had been perceived in the first place.

The GPs showed considerable interest in the findings because we were able to monitor what was happening and plan for the future. They were used to educate other team members about what a social worker could and could not do and I think improved the quality of referrals. I certainly began to receive more information and more counselling work. In this sense it was a valuable exercise.

Unfortunately the research had a largely negative effect on senior management in the Area Office. They were very reluctant to look at, or discuss, the research. They saw Health Centre clients as having lower priority than statutory work, such as report writing. Moreover counselling people with alcohol problems, while advocated by regional policy, was frowned upon locally and was usually dealt with by referral to recommended voluntary agencies. The position improved after the regional restructuring which resulted in a new area manager and senior social worker being appointed who were both interested in, and positive about, the research.

I hope that by publishing this data social work managers may see that health-based social work often reaches very vulnerable clients who would not otherwise get the advice or support they require. It provides a link with the community which may reduce stigma so that in time both the client and the medical professional may come to appreciate social workers in other locations. Perhaps it will also encourage serious thought on the amount of autonomy required by social workers in Health Centres in order to provide an appropriate service. While there continue to be problems, I firmly believe that the Health Centre is the only effective means of providing a truly preventative social work service.

References

1. Sheppard, M. 'You're Not Listening' *Community Care*. 3.9.1987, 23-24.

2. Jenkins, M.E. 'The Attachment of Social Workers to GP Practices.' Research Section, Mid Glamorgan County Council, 1978.

3. Huntington, J. *Social Work and General Medical Practice*. George Allen and Unwin, London, 1981.

4. Huntington, J. *'Social Work and Primary Health Care.'* (Unpublished Report). April 1984.

5. Corney, R.H. 'Social Work in General Practice'. In Lishman, J. (ed.) *Collaboration and Conflict: Working with Others*. Research Highlights, No.7, Aberdeen University, 1983.

6. Corney, R.H., and Bowen, B.A. 'Referrals to Social Workers'. In Clare, A.W., and Corney, R.H. (eds.) *Social Work and Primary Health Care*. Academic Press, 1982, 31-43.

7. Goldberg, E.M., and Neill, J.E. *Social Work in General Practice*. George Allen and Unwin, London, 1972.

8. McLaren, P., and McLean, S. 'Glen Street Area Office Six Months Referral Study Nov. 1980 - April 1981.' Unpublished Report for Strathclyde Region Department of Social Work, Renfrew Division.

9. Winny, J., and Corney R.H. 'The Case for GP Attachments' *Community Care*. 1.7.1982, 18-19.

10. Berne, E. *The Games People Play*. Penguin, 1962.

11. Winny, J., and Rushton, A. 'Social Work in a Health Centre' *Health and Social Service Journal*. 6,3, 1981, 257-259.

12. Reynolds, D.A. 'Healthy Mix' *Community Care*. 13.3.1980, 44-46.

Acknowledgement

I should like to express my thanks to the British Association of Social Workers' Educational Trust for awarding me the Anne Cummins Memorial Scholarship which enabled me to complete this study, to Moira Leitch, then Principal Officer (Health) with Strathclyde Region who encouraged me to apply for the scholarship but above all who greeted my efforts with enthusiasm, and to Jill Ford who has patiently edited this manuscript.

Appendix I - S.R.C. S.W.D. Referral Analysis

Form SW/RR
02/82

551048

S.R.C. S.W.D. REFERRAL ANALYSIS

Transaction Type | Referral Year | Referral Month | Area Team | Ref. Method | Post Code | Reason(s) for Referral | Allocation | Sex/Ref. Status | Age Band | Worker | Marital Status | Benefit | Living Group

Local Opinion Boxes: A | B | C | D

WORK/REFERRAL STATUS

male/known	01
male/unknown	02
female/known	03
female/unknown	04

BAND

0-4	05
5-11	06
12-16	07
17-20	08
21-30	09
31-40	10
41-50	11
51-60	
61-64	
65-74	
over 75	

MARITAL STATUS

married
divorced
widowed
separated
single
co-habitee
child

LIVING GROUP

Family group with child(ren) including 1 or more under fives	01
Family group with child(ren) under 17 but none under 5	02
Single parent household with child(ren) including 1 or more under 5	03
Single parent household with child(ren) under 17 but none under 5	04
Family with no children	05
1 person household—not pensioner	06
1 person pensioner	07
2 persons pensioner	08
Other private household	09
Residential accommodation	10
Other	11

REFERRER

Self	01	Fuel authorities	12
Relative/friend/neighbour	02	Police	13
G.P.	03	Sheriff Court	14
Health Visitor/nurse	04	District Court	15
Other health personnel	05	Reporter	16
Hospital social worker	06	Standby	17
Social work staff outwith Area Office	07	Voluntary agency	18
Housing Department	08	Other	19
Education Dept./School	09		
Other local authority Dept.	10		
D.H.S.S.	11		

REFERRAL METHOD

Telephone	1
Caller	2
Letter	3
Automatic Notification	4
Other	5

REASON FOR REFERRAL

Financial/Material	01
D.H.S.S. Problem Fares/destitution	02
Rent Problems	03
School Uniform	04
Gas	05
S.S.E.B.	06
Housing	10
Homelessness Single	11
Homelessness Family	12
Anti Social Behaviour	13
Re-housing	14
Dampness	15
Repairs	16
Furniture	17
Removal	18
Alcohol/Drug Abuse	20
Alcohol Related Problem	21
Solvent Abuse	22
Drug Abuse	23
Offence Related problems	30
Parole	31
Aftercare	32
Police Warning	33
FSO	34
Probation	35
CSO	36
Request for report/assessment	40
Panel	41
Court	42
Means Enquiry Report	43
Matrimonial proceedings	44
Child minding	45
Adoption	46
Fostering	47
Child related	50
Child abuse	51
Child neglect	52
Child offence	53
Child/parent relationship	54
Truancy	55
Family Social Relationship	60
Marital breakdown	61
Spouse assault	62
Unstable relationship	63
Problem relating to mental handicap	70
Social isolation	71
Mobility	72
Personal care/domestic problem	73
Holiday	74
Problem relating to mental health	75
Psychosis, i.e. schizophrenia	76
Neurosis, i.e. depression	77
Other mental illness not defined	78
Problems relating to physical handicap	80
Social isolation	81
Mobility	82
Personal Care/domestic problems	83
Problems relating to the elderly	90
Social isolation	91
Mobility	92
Personal care/domestic problems	93
Senile dementia	94
Part III Ass	95
Gen Ass	96
Holiday	97

ALLOCATION

Noted/no further action	01
Information/advice/counselling/advocacy and no further action	02
Financial/material assistance and no further action	03
Referral to home help service	04
Referral to OT department	05
Allocated as a short term case	06
Allocated as a long term case	07
Allocated to a senior social worker	08
Admission to care	09
Other	10

WORKER

Intake/duty	1
Long term	3
Senior	4
Admin. worker	5
O.T.	6
Home Help	7
Welfare Rights Officer	8
Community Worker	9
Other	

BENEFIT RECEIPT

Not known	0
No State Benefit	1
Unemployment Benefit	2
Supplementary Benefit	3
Sick/Invalidity Benefit	4
Retirement Pension	5
Widows Pension	6
Ind. Injury Benefit	7
Non-contributory Dis. Pension	8
Child	9

Counselling Elderly People with Mental Health Problems

John Carpenter

Introduction

This chapter describes a project for elderly people with mental health problems. The project arose out of a review of patients referred to a psychiatric day hospital in Weston-super-Mare. A new assessment procedure had been introduced and all new patients were seen together with any friends and family, by a multi-disciplinary team. The assessment was particularly concerned with the psychological, social and relationship problems which had precipitated the initial referral for psychiatric help and which continued to influence the patients' lives.

Approximately one-quarter of the patients assessed were between sixty and seventy-five years of age. A number of striking features about this group were noted: first, that they had been reluctant users of psychiatric services initially and had not been keen to see a psychiatrist or go into hospital; second, with the benefit of hindsight, they considered that the help had come too late. Most had little difficulty in answering the question: 'When did this all start?' Typically, they described some difficult or tragic event in their lives such as a serious illness, breakdown in family relationships or the death of a spouse which had taken place a year or so before. They had felt unable to discuss these concerns with anyone, their worries had increased to the point of psychiatric breakdown when they had been referred, often with a sense of shame, for treatment. The treatment itself had tended to focus on the symptoms of anxiety or depression and was primarily medication. With very few exceptions, these patients welcomed the alternative approach to assessment and help offered by the day hospital staff, often remarking that they wished they had had this assistance a long time ago. The project to be described here was designed to explore the feasibility of providing help to elderly people at an earlier stage of their problems. The aim of the project will be outlined, the methods described and the results presented and discussed in the light of other research reports. But first I will note some evidence concerning the psychological problems of elderly people.

Elderly people and psychological problems

Contrary to most assumptions, elderly people are far more likely to suffer from functional psychiatric disorders like depression than from organic brain syndromes (the dementias). Indeed, functional disorders were found by Kay and colleagues[1] in one in three persons aged sixty-five years and over. (The figure for dementias is one in ten). More than half these disorders were classified as 'neurotic' and though some were judged severe, the patients were rarely receiving treatment.

Elderly people consult their general practitioner more than any other age group. A rate of 180 consultations per 1,000 in two weeks had been reported and although less than ten per cent of these contacts were explicitly recognised to be due to 'mental illness', it is likely that mental health problems contributed to, or were associated with, many more. Relatively few elderly patients are referred to psychiatrists nut they nevertheless account for one-quarter of all admissions to psychiatric hospitals.[2]

Unfortunately, there is some evidence that admission to psychiatric hospital is bad for the health of elderly people with both functional and organic disorders. A significant mortality rate between thirty-five and sixty per cent at the end of a year's follow-up has been reported.[3,4]

Thus there would appear to be a large number of elderly people who are in contact with their general practitioners whose psychological problems are not either recognised or treated until it is too late to prevent hospitalisation and its attendant consequences.

Murphy[5] has demonstrated a strong association between severe life events, major social difficulties, poor physical health and the onset of depression. (Depression is the most common diagnosis in referrals to psychogeriatric services). In a study based on Brown and Harris' psycho-social model of depression,[6] she surveyed elderly patients referred to a psychiatric service and a community sample, some of whom experienced an onset of depression during the study. People experiencing depression were more likely to have experienced a severe life event such as bereavement, life threatening illness or a major negative revelation concerning someone close, major personal illness, financial or material loss and enforced change of residence. Similarly, they were more likely to have experienced major social difficulties especially in family and marital relationships, housing and financial problems. Studies such as this confirm the statements of Bowlby and Parkes concerning the importance of loss, and of Brody concerning the relevance of family problems in the development of psychiatric illness in elderly people.[7,8,9]

The relationship between physical illness and mental health problems is of considerable significance in elderly people. Poor physical health is an obvious source of mental stress, but in addition it may 'mask' psychological problems. For example, a patient who presents diffuse and non-specific physical symptoms against a background of anorexia, weight loss and lack of sleep could be suffering from a malignant illness and/or be depressed.[10] Similarly, facial pain in women and persistent neck pain in men are frequently indications of depression but may not be recognised as such by the general practitioner, especially if the patient denies any other physical symptoms of depression. It appears that such patients are a high suicide risk.[10] On the other hand, depression is a common side effect of drugs given for the treatment of physical disease: the incidence of adverse reactions increases with age, elderly people are given more drugs of all kinds than younger people and make more mistakes in taking them. The general practitioners' role in diagnosing physical and psychological problems in elderly people is of obvious importance.

Aims of the project

Given the evidence that elderly people with psychological problems were likely to be in contact with their general practitioner, it was decided to establish the project in a primary health care setting. The project would offer a counselling service to elderly people identified by their general practitioner as having suffered a severe life event in the context of social difficulties and thus being at risk of psychiatric illness. The project was designed as a piece of 'action' research in which the feasibility of a preventative approach would be explored. In other words, it would aim to discover the practical requirements and means of operation and not simply to measure the effectiveness or otherwise of a method of intervention. More particularly, it aimed to establish:

- The necessary practical arrangements
- Whether general practitioners could identify appropriate clients
- Whether these clients were being helped by other agencies and if so, what distinctive contribution could be made by the project
- Would prospective clients agree to meet a counsellor?
- What problems and needs do the clients have?
- What methods of psychological and social intervention were appropriate?
- What liaison with the general practitioners was necessary?
- How many clients would be referred and how much counsellor time was required?
- The effectiveness of the service for each client.

The answers to these questions would indicate not only whether or not the project was feasible and effective but also how the service could be replicated, by whom and with what resources.

Establishing the project

I decided to offer one session (morning or afternoon) of counselling to a group practice of general practitioners. The introductory letter drew on the evidence presented above to make a case for a trial project. The practice was asked to make a room available and to identify and refer suitable patients. These were defined as being: over sixty years of age, having psychological (including psychiatric) problems and relationship problems, and not having been in contact with psychiatric services for the last two years. The reason for this last condition was that the project was intended to be preventative and not to take over or duplicate existing services.

The first practice approached expressed interest but was unable to offer a suitable interviewing room - a partitioned section of the general waiting area hardly offered significant guarantee of confidentiality and the alternative of an examination room complete with couch did not promise the right ambience! That there did not seem to be sufficient will to overcome this obstacle was taken by me as an indication of lukewarm commitment.

A second practice was much more welcoming. One of the partners' rooms would always be available on the morning I asked for, so long as I did not mind changing occasionally in order to accommodate the duty rota, holiday cover and hospital responsibilities. I attended a meeting of the partners in order to describe the project more fully, answer questions about the kind of referrals I was looking for, consider practical arrangements and discuss liaison and confidentiality.

It was agreed that referrals should be made on a standard form rather than by letter or word of mouth. There were a number of reasons for this: first, a form which asks the referee to indicate the reason for referral by ticking a box provides a straightforward check of eligibility - which problems can be considered and which not (i.e. the project does offer counselling for marital problems but not assessment for a place in a local authority home). Second, the form requires the referee to consider carefully why he or she is making the referral and not simply to suggest that a potential client has 'lots of problems - see what you can do to help'. Third, the form can ask for information which might or might not be covered in a general practitioner's letter, information such as: details of spouse, family and other significant people; the involvement of other agencies; and about the relationship between the general practitioner and the potential client. The actual form used in the project is shown in Appendix 1.

Other practical arrangements made included using the practice secretaries and receptionists to send invitation letters and to deal with clients in exactly the same way as the users of general medical services. In other words, there would be nothing to distinguish a client coming to the project from any visit to the doctor - except the greater length of time available. It was also agreed that the clients would be referred to a 'counsellor' on the grounds that the use of the term 'social worker' could cause confusion with district or hospital social workers.

Perhaps surprisingly, the partners offered open access to their patients' medical records and proposed that no details of the content of the counselling should be included in the notes, unless there was explicit agreement with the client that this could serve a specific purpose. All that would be required were indications that a client was being seen for counselling and when the sessions had finished. It was further agreed with the social work manager that similar details only were required for the local authority's records. Finally, I offered details of where I could be contacted during the working week so that if necessary, any crisis which occurred in the lives of clients in the project could be discussed immediately and before my next scheduled visit to the surgery.

Operation

I ran the project for three years from 1984 to 1987 and have analysed the 54 cases which were referred and closed during that time. An earlier evaluation was made after the first fifteen months when it was decided that the project should continue and, if possible, be extended to other surgeries. This has now been done and the original project has also been handed over to another social worker. The results and discussion which follow refer to the first three years only. The analysis is based on the initial referral form, a case review system and general practitioner assessment, to be described below, and three project review meetings with the partners at different stages.

Practical arrangements

There were no difficulties with the practical arrangements discussed at the beginning of the project and described above. The project made few demands on secretarial time: the secretaries used a pro-forma letter of invitation and follow-up appointments were made in the surgery's appointments book; the receptionists agreed to telephone me in advance with any notice of cancellations and to make substitute appointments for anyone on the 'waiting list'. The only costs to the surgery were use of the telephone to contact clients or agencies on their behalf and liberal supplies of coffee!

Referrals

The total number of patients on the practice list on 7th May 1986 classified by age and sex was as follows:

Total Patients = 10,582
Number of Patients over sixty = 2,662 (33.6%)

The high proportion of elderly people is typical of a seaside retirement town. They were served by four full-time male and one part-time female general practitioners. The 'target group' for the project was people over sixty and, in practice, under eighty years of age, since the very elderly group of patients were much less mobile and living predominantly in sheltered housing or homes. The number of patients referred by age and sex and the numbers on the list are shown in Table 1.

TABLE 1
Age and sex distribution of cases referred and closed over three years

Number of patients

Age		Referred	On list	Percentage referred
60-74	Female	35	1017	3.4
	Male	4	782	0.5
	Total	39	1799	2.2
74-81	Female	13	326	4.0
	Male	2	176	1.1
	Total	15	502	3.0
	Grand Total	54	2301	2.4

It can be seen from Table 1 that the number of patients referred to the project was a small proportion of the patients on the list and that strikingly few men were referred (six out of fifty-four, or eleven per cent). The possible reasons for these facts will be discussed later.

There was also a marked difference in the rate of referral between the partners: the part-time female general practitioner referred exactly one half the number of clients to the project although only ten per cent of the patients were on her 'personal' list. A further twenty-five per cent of the cases were referred by the youngest male partner who had a similarly small personal list. The two most senior partners referred only eight patients between them. Possible explanations for these variations will be considered later.

The total number of referrals made during the three years (i.e. the fifty-four cases analysed here plus cases which remained open) represented an average of a little over twenty per year. Between three and five clients were seen for up to one hour each during the morning session of three hours. With these small numbers there was a delicate balance between too much and too little work and this varied during the course of the three years. Three new referrals in one week could easily overload the project, particularly if they coincided with annual leave. At other times in the early months, the closure of a few cases and a drought in referrals meant that it was necessary to prompt partners. Overall, the one session per week proved adequate to the number of elderly people referred.

Marital status and living arrangement

The majority of clients were widowed and/or living alone:

Marital Status	**Living Arrangement**
Single 5 (9%)	Alone 34 (63%)
Married 14 (26%)	With spouse/cohabitee 16 (29%)
Widowed 31 (57%)	With friend 2 (4%)
Separated 2 (4%)	Private residential home 2 (4%)
Divorced 2 (4%)	

It is worth noting that although sixty-three per cent are designated as 'living alone', at least two-thirds of these people had regular contact with other members of their family. Whilst many of these contacts were helpful and supportive, there were many instances of difficulties in family relationships which contributed towards poor adjustment to change.

Involvement with other agencies

Other agencies were very rarely involved with clients in the project. One was in regular contact with a health visitor, another with a district nurse, one with a hospital social worker and one with a specialist social worker for people with a visual handicap. Six were in contact with a hospital doctor for in-patient or out-patient care.

Reason for referral

All the fifty-four cases analysed here were considered appropriate in the sense that they met the referral criteria. Two other referrals of 'under-age' people were made during this period and were taken on after assessment of their particular needs; they were however excluded from this study. In twenty-three cases more than one reason was given for the referral. The reasons are summarised in Table 2.

TABLE 2
Reasons for referral to Project by General Practitioner

Difficulties in adjusting to loss or change (including bereavement)	33
Marital problems	8
Family problems	8
Difficulties in coping with ill health	16
Psychosomatic problems	10
Dying spouse	2
Total	77

Methods of work

The project was monitored using a *case review system* derived from a study of mental health social work by Fisher and his colleagues.[11] This was in turn derived from the work of Goldberg and Warburton[12] and involves a review of all cases open during the previous three months. The review requires an assessment of the severity of mental/emotional disturbance and of impairment of social/emotional functioning in terms of interpersonal relationships and personal care. It asks for a concise description of the current situation and for changes since the last review. There is a check list on which to indicate the focus of work and the outcome of cases closed during the review period. The review form used in the project is included as Appendix 2.

This case review system of monitoring has a number of advantages for practitioners, not least its ease of operation; the review is straightforward but it also stimulates reflection and planning; in addition, all cases are reviewed at the same time, so a comprehensive set of information can be gathered in the space of a few minutes. Also, the system can include clients as active participants in the review.[13] In this project, separate review appointments were made three months after the case was closed in which the clients' opinions were sought in completing the form.

Regarding the aims of the project, the case review made it possible to answer the questions concerning the clients' problems and needs, the methods of psychological social intervention which were necessary, the amount of time necessary and an indication of the outcome in each case. I will first summarise the reviews and then discuss some illustrative case examples.

Severity of mental/emotional disturbance

Following Fisher et al's case review system[11] this was assessed in terms of 'impaired perception of reality' and 'inappropriate feelings'. Assessment at first interview showed the former to be very unusual, with only three clients being judged as having slightly distorted perceptions. These three seemed to be mildly paranoid, out this was easily explicable in terms of their recent experiences. Nobody was considered seriously confused or psychotic. Bereavement reactions were excluded from this analysis since hallucinations and depression are normal reactions. Three quarters of the remaining clients were assessed as having slight or marked inappropriate feelings including anxiety, hopelessness and worthlessness.

Impairment of social/emotional functioning

Interpersonal family relationships were at least strained (twenty-five per cent) or beginning to break down (thirty-five per cent) and in fifteen per cent of cases had completely broken down. In wider social relationships, the problems were apparently less severe and clients were more likely to report loneliness and isolation than arguments and disputes. In terms of personal care, a minority (thirty-five per cent) had periods of self-neglect - usually not eating adequately or letting their appearance go somewhat.

Focus of work

The focus of work with each client changed as problems were resolved and/or new ones appeared. In the following analysis, the primary focus during the previous three months as indicated on 160 review forms is shown. It is important to stress that the primary focus was never the sole focus and also that longer term work will be overestimated compared to short-term work because more review forms will have been completed. Nevertheless, this analysis does give a crude estimate of the balance of work.

TABLE 3

Primary focus of counselling

Grief counselling	38
(Morbid) grief therapy	12
Family and marital relationships	50
Conjoint marital therapy	14
Relationships with others	14
Self-management	22
Information/advice	10

1. Grief counselling

Well over half of the referrals to the project concerned difficulties in adjusting to loss and change. As expected, many of these followed the bereavement of a spouse but it should not be assumed that recent widows and widowers were referred routinely. Rather, by agreement, the partners referred only those cases where the bereavement reaction seemed complicated, either when it seemed unusually intense or, more usually, when the process had become stuck and mourning was not taking place. Such complications are more likely when certain 'risk factors' are present. These include: a painful or mismanaged death; a high degree of dependence on, or an ambivalent relationship with, the dead partner; physical disability or illness; and lack of family support.[14] In particular, elderly people bereaved of their spouse after a lengthy illness do less well than those bereaved after a short fatal illness.[15]

The loss of the relationship with the dead partner is, of course, not the only change which takes place after death. Those patients referred to the project were more likely to have experienced a number of changes, as the following case illustrates:

> *Mrs A* (aged seventy-five) was referred nine months after her husband's death and subsequent move from her house in the country to a flat in town. Shortly after her move she had had a coronary and was admitted to hospital. To make matters worse, following her discharge she had suffered a small stroke which had left her with visual problems. Mrs A had great difficulty in accepting her husband's death and, indeed, had not talked about him at all with her family who were concerned not to distress her for fear that this might provoke another heart attack.
>
> Mrs A was brought to the first session by one of her daughters and encouraged to 'tell her story'. Slowly and hesitantly at first, she explained what had happened, how she had nursed him during a long illness, the shock when he did eventually die and the tremendous support her family had been in finding another place to live. As she talked amid many tears, it became apparent that her daughter too had not mourned her father and that the family's concern with practical arrangements for 'Mother' rather than for her emotional needs had inadvertently disabled her from the normal grieving process. Further, in their concern to look after her, they had taken away all her control over her life - this from a woman who had brought up five children, ran a home and nursed a sick man for many years.
>
> Over the course of the next six sessions, in which two of the other daughters also became involved, Mrs A and her children were able to begin mourning Mr A. Mrs A had also to mourn the loss of her home, her role as someone who cared for others, the loss of her good health and the loss of her independence. She was not sufficiently well to live on her own in the flat and moved into a residential home - into which she was allowed to bring her own furniture and to arrange it in the way she wanted. Her children had been able to take the message that to express their feelings was safe, both for themselves and their mother.

Knowing how someone grieved a previous loss is particularly useful, as in the following example:

> *Mrs B* (aged 64) had lost her second husband suddenly whilst they were on holiday 'wintering' in Spain. He had had a heart attack and had been taken by ambulance to hospital where he died before Mrs B, following on behind in a taxi which had broken down, had been able to reach him. The referring general practitioner, who was not, incidentally, her regular doctor, had asked about Mrs B's first husband and her response to his death. It emerged that she had not mourned at the time but, as the medical records confirmed, she had been thrice admitted to psychiatric hospital, receiving anti-depressants and ECT.

> In Mrs B's case I had to take an active and forceful approach in order to provoke her mourning: a break-through came when her daughter-in-law, whom I had recruited as a 'co-therapist', took her to the crematorium which she had previously been quite unable to visit.

Of course not all loss is death:

> *Mrs C* (aged sixty-seven), a widow, was referred with acute, persistent toothache for which the dental hospital could find no adequate physical explanation. She only came at her general practitioner's insistence, stating that she didn't see how counselling could possibly help. She was certainly very angry and upset, feeling that she had been let down by 'everybody' - especially the dental hospital and her doctor. After a while, she revealed that the people she was really angry with were her daughter and son-in-law who had announced quite unexpectedly that they and their children were emigrating to Australia in one month's time. Her existence revolved around her family, she had made little life for herself in Weston-super-Mare and had only moved there following her husband's death in order to be with them. Their announcement had left her literally speechless - and the ache in her mouth seemed understandable as a straightforward psycho-somatic reaction. She had not seen them since.

> With help, Mrs C re-established contact with her family, engaged in some anticipatory grieving and managed to say good-bye at the airport.

2. Grief therapy

In the examples discussed above, the process of grieving had become blocked and the counsellors' task was to set it going again. Whilst accepting that there is a continuous relationship between normal and abnormal grief (often referred to as pathological, morbid or unresolved grief), Worden[16] nevertheless makes a distinction between the two in terms of the intensity and duration of the reaction. He treats as abnormal reactions which are 'chronic', 'delayed', 'exaggerated' or 'masked'. Dealing with chronic or exaggerated grief reactions is relatively straightforward since they are easily recognised: the counsellor and client can assess together which of the tasks of mourning have not been completed and why, and an appropriate intervention made. Delayed or masked grief reactions are less obvious but, as the following two examples illustrate, once recognised can be successfully resolved.

> *Mrs D* (aged sixty-six) was referred some months after the death of her second husband. She was surprised by the intensity of her reaction because she freely admitted she had not cared much for him and had deeply resented having to nurse him through blindness and incontinence before he died. Her reaction certainly seemed to be out of proportion to her attachment to him, even allowing for a degree of ambivalence. Through the counselling sessions we established that she was in delayed grief for her first husband who had died forty-two years earlier. She descried him as a romantic music hall conductor. He had died of throat cancer quite unexpectedly, leaving her with a ten week old baby. In an apparent search for stability after her exciting but hazardous first marriage, she had married a divorcee twenty years older who was singularly dull by comparison. She had had neither the time nor the opportunity to mourn her first husband, whose loss she now felt all the more intensely.

Grief is often 'masked' by physical symptoms. The most dramatic example seen on the project was Mrs E (aged 81) who was referred with a variety of problems, thought by the general practitioner to be psychosomatic.

> *Mrs E*'s medical file was 4 inches thick! It detailed numerous physical examinations by a complete range of medical and surgical specialists who, in spite of a variety of tests and exploratory operations, had never managed to find anything of real significance. Some years previously, she had been referred to a psychiatrist who had pronounced her a 'well known hypochondriac' and sent her back to her general practitioner. On entering the office, she remarked: 'I don't know why I've come to see you'. 'Yes, I gather you've been to see rather a lot of people', I said, gesturing at her file on the desk. 'Yes, ever since my husband died', she replied.

As her story unfolded it became clear that, although she talked as if it were yesterday, she was referring to the first of three husbands who had died twenty years previously. Perhaps of greatest significance was the revelation, which until then she had not even recognised herself, that on the day he died, her husband had given a clear indication that he was going to divorce her. Sharing this revelation, and the hurt and anger she felt, removed the block to her mourning and, in almost dramatic fashion, the physical pain she felt too. After six sessions she pronounced that she had 'never felt better - barring a spot of arthritis which is normal at my age'.

The goals and procedures for grief therapy have been outlined by Worden[16] who recommends a contracted, focussed approach. He suggests reviving memories, both positive and negative and dealing with the emotion or lack of it, which they stimulate. I would agree with his contention that grief therapy demands a high degree of skill and emotional resilience on the part of the worker, beyond that usually expected for grief counselling.

3. Family and marital relationships

Although problems in marital and family relationships were not very often cited as the reason for referral (see Table 2), they were nevertheless, the most frequent primary focus of work (Table 3). There are two possible explanations for this fact. First, work begun with a focus on another problem such as grieving often developed a primary concern for family relationships (for example in the case of Mrs C described above). Second, the reason for referral given by the general practitioner was not always seen by the client as a full and accurate description of his or her situation.

For example, *Mrs F* (aged sixty-nine) was referred because she was unhappy about her recent move to Weston-super-Mare (i.e. for difficulties in adjusting to change). However, it turned out that this move had been the fourth move in the seven years since her husband's retirement and he was refusing to entertain the idea of a fifth! After discussion, Mrs F acknowledged that yet another move would not solve her problems, which were not to do with her liking or disliking a particular house or area, but rather with the unsatisfactory nature of her relationship with her husband. She described herself as his 'slave' - a position she had held ever since he had returned disabled from the War. Not only had she nursed him daily but she had also obeyed his every wish, 'waiting on him hand and foot'. She had now 'rebelled' and intended, now that he had retired, to have her way for a change.

Mrs F agreed to let me meet her husband, on his own in the first instance and then in two joint sessions. He insisted that he had no intention of moving and expressed irritation at the way his wife kept 'fussing' over him. He wanted to enjoy his retirement by developing his own interests, just as she was free to develop hers. After much discussion and an experimental visit to her daughter in London, she was persuaded that he was not nearly so dependent on her as she thought - he didn't need a slave any longer. Indeed, once she had stopped being his slave they discovered that they could also be friends and instituted a weekly lunch out together when they could enjoy each other's company and which she didn't have to cook.

In many cases of family relationship problems, however, it was not possible to bring the parties together, either because they were reluctant to attend, or more often, because they lived too far away. It was still possible to effect change in relationships by maintaining a systematic perspective, as the following case illustrates.

Mrs G (aged seventy-four) suffered from a number of physical problems which she recognised appeared when she was under stress. She associated this stress with her elder unmarried daughter (aged forty-two) who was still dependent on her for emotional and financial support, although she lived many miles away. Mrs G resented this dependence but found it impossible to reject any of her requests.

Over the course of eight sessions, Mrs G was encouraged to lay down some rules for both her daughters and establish that she was not an endless source of money. She rehearsed various tactics for dealing with visits and phone calls in role-play with me. The daughter continued to be unsettled, but Mrs G could keep her problems at an appropriate distance. Eventually she even went on a trip to Canada, telling her daughter that she should take this as a vote of confidence in her ability to cope on her own!

4. Relationships with others

In many cases a focus on relationships with other people who were not family members developed from earlier work on different issues.

For example, *Mr H* (aged eighty-seven) asked to see me again one year after the conclusion of some bereavement counselling. This time he was troubled about other people living in the residential home with him. He did not believe that the management would be sympathetic to his complaints. In three subsequent sessions, we considered ways of tackling these problems which were overcome in large part when Mr H convinced the manager to let him change rooms.

5. Self-management/information and advice

Self-management refers to a focus on more straightforward aspects of daily life, including managing financial affairs, developing social activities and encouraging clients to look after themselves whilst living alone for the first time. In some cases only information and advice were necessary, whilst in others, I acted as advocate for the client with the DHSS, housing department and fuel services. In one case I agreed to speak to the referring general practitioner on the client's behalf!

Evaluation

As described above, a case review system was used to monitor the project and a joint assessment with each client was made at a follow-up interview approximately three months after the case was closed. This joint assessment was not possible in cases where the client withdrew, left the area or died and also in those cases (four) where an initial contact was not achieved. In all the other cases a follow-up review took place; if the client did not come to the interview I made contact by telephone and in two cases received replies to letters.

The referring general practitioners also completed a case summary sheet having consulted the patient's medical notes. This summary asked for information on the patient's surgery attendance concerning the referred or related problems. It also asked for an assessment of the results of the counselling and left space for additional comments. The results of these evaluations are shown in Table 4.

It should be acknowledged that such assessments are relatively crude. Nevertheless, the social work assessment was made with reference to the individual clients and were reasonably consistent with the general practitioner's independent assessment overall, although the degree of consistency is over-emphasised in the table. This is because some cases were rated quite differently. For example, some cases in which I had considered aims could not be effected were rated as partial success by the general practitioners and vice versa; similarly there was not always consensus about the extent to which aims had been achieved. This is hardly surprising since the aims themselves were not agreed between referrer and counsellor and it would not be reasonable to assume that they were the same.

TABLE 4
Outcome of counselling

	Social Work Assessment	General Practitioner Assessment
Aims achieved	23 ⎤	29 ⎤
Aims partially achieved	11 ⎦ 34	13 ⎦ 42
Aims cannot be effected	7 ⎤	6 ⎤
Client withdrew	7 ⎦ 14	- ⎦ 6
Aims partially or wholly achieved	69%	85%
Client died	1	1
Initial contact not achieved	4	4
TOTAL	54	54

Number of sessions

There was considerable variation in the number of sessions involving clients in the project. Most contacts were for between four and nine sessions with one in five clients becoming relatively long-term (sixteen to twenty sessions could easily spread over a year). These long term clients included two couples with intractable marital problems and eight individuals who were relatively isolated with few friends and no social supports. Four of these had severe difficulty in adjusting to bereavement and the other four had long-term relationship and social problems, including poor accommodation and shortage of money.

Eight clients who had between one and three sessions included four who withdrew and four for whom the aims of counselling were achieved. Their personal resources tended to be greater and, in the main, required reassurance that they were tackling their problems correctly. Four clients who did not come had all been referred by the same partner. In two cases it seems that they simply thought they could manage on their own. The other two seemed to have experienced the referral as a rejection by their doctor. This supposition is confirmed by the observation that this doctor reported some difficulty in making referrals of patients with whom she had a good relationship. I will comment further on this issue in the final section.

Discussion

The project described in this paper is best described as a part-time attachment scheme, in that I took referrals from the general practice and used the practice premises.[18] In terms of effective collaboration, attachment schemes are claimed to be superior to liaison schemes (in which the social worker visits the practice regularly to collect referrals and discuss cases).[19,20] In attachment schemes, social workers are better able to 'educate' their medical colleagues to recognise their skills and to make appropriate referrals. This may be especially true for clients with psychological problems who are apparently more likely to be referred once the social worker has become known and trusted and, perhaps, 'earned' this trust through effective 'bread and butter' practical work.[21,22] In this context, it is perhaps surprising that the general practitioners in this project were ready, from the beginning, to accept a social worker's expertise in counselling people with mental health problems and, further, that all the referrals were appropriate. However, I did present myself as a member of the local multi-disciplinary mental health team and not as a district social worker and so relevant expertise was assumed. This expertise was presumably confirmed by the initial presentation of the project brief and the detailed discussion about the types of referral sought. I have no doubt that the referral form itself helped shape the kind of referrals made. The detailed preliminary discussions about referrals and practical arrangements, and the subsequent reviews were certainly important in ensuring the success of the project and in avoiding the pitfalls of poor co-operation and inappropriate referrals described in earlier surveys.[20,23]

Referrals

The project demonstrated that the general practitioners *could* identify patients who met the project criteria, who were therefore 'at risk' of serious psychological problems and subsequently of psychiatric referral and possible hospital admission. In a number of cases, the general practitioners acknowledged that they had referred to the project as an alternative to referral to a psychiatrist; in others, they apparently assumed that such a referral would be necessary if there was no improvement in the patient's life. Nevertheless, it seems likely that the existence of the project made *early* referral for specialist help more likely; the partners were 'on the look out' for suitable cases and their sensitivity was raised. None of the referrals were considered trivial, the partners showed discrimination (notably in relation to the severity of bereavement reactions) and so this increased sensitivity did not 'create' new clients.

Whilst the doctors *did* identify a group of elderly people in need, it is highly improbable that they identified *all* possible clients. That they did not is strongly suggested by two facts: the very small number of men referred; and the variation between partners. There is no evidence that elderly men's psychological health is so much better than women's which could account for the gross discrepancy in rates of referral (see Table 1). The only possible explanations are: males' reticence in talking about emotional matters (which is probably stronger in old age); and doctors' lack of sensitivity to men's psychological problems (which is the other side of the coin).

The variation between partners in the number of referrals each made can be explained by a number of factors.[24] These include: the individual doctor's sensitivity; his or her attitude to the project; the extent to which he or she engaged in counselling patients; and the wishes of the patients themselves. Thus, while all the partners were positive about the project, there were different degrees of enthusiasm evident in, for example, the speed with which forms were completed. One partner liked to do his own counselling and reported that his patients did not want to leave him - they apparently implied that he was rejecting them. Indeed, the patients he did refer were those with whom he was having difficulty!

The most important factors in the variation in referral rate were almost certainly the doctors' sensitivities and their patients' perceptions of their sensitivity and likely interest. Thus, it was clear that a number of patients had chosen to go and see the one female doctor in the practice, although she was not their regular doctor. In some instances they would make the reason explicit. For example, in one case the patient is reported to have said:

'I wanted to see someone I could talk to. I didn't want to bother Dr. X with my *feelings*. Of course, he's a wonderful doctor....'

An interesting sidelight on this was provided by the surgery receptionists who remarked that female patients, especially, would ask to see the 'lady doctor' on the grounds that the appointment would be a 'long one' - apparently the female general practitioner was seen as being less busy and as someone whose time was less valuable than her male colleagues.

Unfortunately, no record was kept of the number of patients who declined their doctor's offer of an appointment with me. The impression I gained from talking to the partners was that it may have been as high as one in four. As suggested above, one possible reason, in a long-standing relationship, was the patient's sense of rejection by the doctor on whom they had learnt to depend. Again, in some new cases to the surgery it is possible that patients felt they were being 'palmed off' onto another person before they had got to know their doctor. The four people who did not arrive for their first appointment included two in each category.

The very small number of patients who did not show (eight per cent) contrasts with a generally higher failure rate in out-patient psychiatric departments. A familiar context, with the absence of any stigmatising procedures and no mention of a psychiatrist, no doubt explains the difference.

If we assume that the doctors did not identify all the possible clients and that these clients did not make themselves known through another doctor, it follows that some elderly people, especially men, were not reached by the project. How could they have been found? A number of possibilities are suggested. First, all elderly patients could be screened for psychological problems and risk factors as part of a general health screening.[25] This was, in fact, discussed and planned with the health visitors attached to the practice but the screening programme had to be halted shortly after it was begun when one health visitor left. Second, a notice advertising the service might have been placed in the waiting room. Third, the partners could have been asked explicitly to screen all elderly people who came to the surgery, perhaps by asking them two or three standard 'leading' questions. Finally, occasional case discussions in the practice meeting might have stimulated more referrals, especially if the discussion had been focussed on the psychological needs of men.

The project clearly demonstrated the range of psychological problems of elderly people (see Table 2). There is abundant evidence that these problems are usually overlooked by social workers or, if recognised, are not the focus of social work intervention.[26,27] Most elderly clients who come to the attention of social workers receive advice and information and are put in touch with appropriate forms of practical help.

Short-term, focussed counselling is very unusual, a fact partly explained by elderly people being social workers' least preferred client group[26] and partly by clients being unaware that social workers did counselling.

This project was not designed as a rigorous outcome study but rather as a piece of practitioner research. The assessment of outcome (Table 4) should therefore be treated with caution. However, the assessment was made from three perspectives, the general practitioner, and the client and social worker together. It is probably true that the 'social work assessments' of the clients who withdrew are a little pessimistic (withdrawal was counted as a failure, although the general practitioner considered four cases as being partial successes). Similarly, the extent to which aims were judged achieved may be a little conservative. The 'truth' probably lies somewhere between the two assessments. The 'success' rate was therefore between sixty-nine and eighty-five per cent, the lower figure being comparable to that reported by Corney and Clare[28] in a controlled study of social work with younger depressed women (aged 18-45) in an attachment scheme. It is interesting to note in their study that the clients who gained most benefit were those who had been depressed for some time and who had a poor relationship with spouse or boyfriend. In the project, poor or non-existent close personal relationships were the norm - hence the major focus on grief work and family and marital relationships. Similarly, in most cases the problems were, by Corney and Clare's definition, chronic (three months). The majority of elderly people seen in the project could therefore have been expected to benefit.

The general practitioners were certainly enthusiastic about the project and wrote in support of its continuation after I left. Their comments included:

'It is important to continue the service as I feel it has proved extremely valuable to the patients who have attended.'

'Patients referred here found the time and help invaluable and I feel it has in many instances prevented the formation of chronic psychiatric cases...none of my patients has had anything but praise for the service offered.'

'I found the service extremely helpful...I do feel it has averted many formal requests later for psychiatric help.'

In conclusion, the project has been continued and, following presentation of the initial review to health and social services managers, it has been extended to two other surgeries. It seems reasonable to claim that it demonstrated a successful approach to helping elderly people who, on the basis of existing research evidence, could be considered to be 'at risk' of psychiatric illness. These people were not being helped by other agencies and, in most cases, short-term, focussed counselling was effective. Further, the project is an example of easy collaborative working between general practice and social work which made few demands on the resources of either agency. Finally, it demonstrates an approach to small-scale 'action research', which was effective in influencing local services, that could be applied to other settings and problems.

References

1. Kay, D. et al. 'Old Age Mental Disorders. A Study of Prevalence' *British Journal of Psychiatry.* 110, 1964, 146-158.

2. Jolley, D., and Arie, T. 'Organisation of Psychogeriatric Services' *British Journal of Psychiatry.* 132, 1978, 1-11.

3. Baker, A., and Bryne, R. 'Another Style of Psychogeriatric Service' *British Journal of Psychiatry.* 130, 1977, 123-126.

4. Turner, R., and Sternbeg, M. 'Psychosocial Factors in Elderly People Admitted to a Psychiatric Hospital.' *Age and Ageing*. 7, 1978, 171-177.

5. Murphy, E. 'Social Origins of Depression in Old Age' *British Journal of Psychiatry*. 141, 1982, 135-142.

6. Brown, G., and Harris, T. *Social Origins of Depression*. Tavistock, London, 1978.

7. Bowlby, J. *Attachment and Loss: Loss, Sadness and Depression*. Vol. III. Penguin, Harmondsworth, 1980.

8. Parkes, C.M. 'Bereavement and Mental Illness' *British Journal of Medical Psychology*. 38, 1965,1-26.

9. Brody, E.H. 'The Ageing Family' *Gerontologist*. 6, 1966, 201-206.

10. Evans, J.E. et al. 'The Interaction between Physical and Psychiatric Disease in the Elderly' *Update*. 23, 1986, 265-272.

11. Fisher, M., Newton, C., and Sainsbury, E. *Mental Health Social Work Observed*. Allen and Unwin, London, 1984.

12. Goldberg, E.M., and Warburton, R.W. *Ends and Means in Social Work: The Development and Outcome of a Case Review System for Social Workers*. Allen and Unwin, London, 1979.

13. Goldberg, E.M., and Connelly, N. 'How to Evaluate.' Ch.3 in *The Effectiveness of Social Care for the Elderly: An Overview of Recent and Current Evaluative Research*. Heinemann, London, 1982.

14. Parkes, C.M. 'Bereavement' *British Journal of Psychiatry*. 146, 1985, 11-17.

15. Gerber, I., Rusalem, R., Hannan, B., Battin, D., and Arkin, A. 'Anticipatory Grief and Aged Widows and Widowers' *Journal of Gerontology*. 30, 1985, 225-229.

16. Worden, J.W. *Grief Counselling and Grief Therapy*. Tavistock, London, 1983.

17. Herr, J., and Weakland, J. *Counselling Elders and their Families: Practical Techniques for Applied Gerontology*. Springer, New York, 1979.

18. Corney, R. 'Social Work in General Practice' *Journal of the Royal College of General Practitioners*. 35, 1985, 291-292.

19. Corney, R. 'A Comparative Study of Referrals to a Local Authority Intake Team with a General Practice Attachment Scheme and the Resulting Social Workers' Interventions' *Social Science and Medicine*. 14, 1980, 675-682.

20. Winny, J., and Corney, R. 'The case for General Practice Attachments' *Community Care*. 1.7.1982, 18-19.

21. Forman, J., and Fairbairn, E. *Social Casework in General Practice*. Oxford University Press, London, 1968.

22. Goldberg, E., and Neill, J. *Social Work in General Practice*. Allen and Unwin, London, 1972.

23. Gilchrist, I., Gough, J., and Horsfall-Turner, U. 'Social Work in General Practice' *Journal of the Royal College of General Practitioners*. 28, 1978, 675-686.

24. Goldberg, D., and Huxley, P.M. *Mental Illness in the Community*. Tavistock, London, 1980.

25. Freer, C. 'Geriatric Screening: A Re-appraisal of Preventative Strategies in the Care of the Elderly' *Journal of the Royal College of General Practitioners*. 35, 1985, 288-290.

26. Goldberg, E.M., and Connelly, N. 'Social Work.' Ch.6 in *The Effectiveness of Social Care for the Elderly: An Overview of Recent and Current Evaluative Research*. Heinemann, London, 1982.

27. Fisher, M., Newton, C., and Sainsbury, E. 'The Clients in the Study'. Chapter 4 In *Mental Health Social Work Observed*. Ch.4. Allen and Unwin, London, 1984.

28. Corney, R., and Clare, A. 'The Effectiveness of Attached Social Workers in the Management of Depressed Women in General Practice' *British Journal of Social Work*. 13, 1983, 57-74.

Appendix I

COUNSELLING PROJECT

REFERRAL FORM FOR ASSESSMENT

NAME........................D.o.B..........MARITAL STATUS.........

ADDRESS.....................................TELEPHONE NO.........

SPOUSE

NAME..................ADDRESS (if different from above).........

CHILDREN
          NAME   ADDRESS

     ....
     ....

OTHER SIGNIFICANT PEOPLE (e.g., parents, in-laws, friends,
                         helpful neighbours)

OTHER AGENCIES INVOLVED

__ Health Visitor   __ Social Worker (Hospital) __ Social Worker
                                                     (District)
__ District Nurse   __ Home Help   __ Hospital Doctor

REASON FOR REFERRAL   Please specify

__ Difficulties in adjusting to
   loss or change

__ Marital problems

__ Family problems

__ Psychosomatic problems

__ Difficulties in coping with ill-health

__ Other

Remarks

How long have you known this patient?

How often does he/she attend surgery?

                              Signed ....

                              Date   ....

Appendix II

UNIVERSITY OF BRISTOL / AVON SOCIAL SERVICES DEPARTMENT

<u>COUNSELLING PROJECT FOR ELDERLY PEOPLE: REVIEW FORM</u>

NAME	**REVIEW DATE** ⬚⬚⬚⬚⬚⬚
Code **SEVERITY OF MENTAL/EMOTIONAL DISTURBANCE** 1 None. 2 Slight. 3 Marked. 4. Severe. (a) Impaired Perception of Reality ☐ (b) Inappropriate feelings ☐	**DESCRIBE PRESENT SITUATION**
Code **IMPAIRMENT OF SOCIAL/EMOTIONAL FUNCTIONING** 1 None. 2 Slight. 3 Marked. 4 Severe (a) Interpersonal (family) ☐ (b) Interpersonal (in wider social relationships) ☐ (c) Personal care ☐	**DESCRIBE CHANGES**

FOCUS OF THERAPEUTIC ACTIVITY
 	
(1) Grief counselling ☐
(2) (Morbid) grief therapy ☐
(3) Family relationships ☐
(4) Relationships with others ☐
(5) Self-management ☐
(6) Information/Advice ☐
 	
Code **PRIMARY FOCUS** ☐
	OPEN CASES
	
	No sessions so far: ☐
	Estimated number of
	  future sessions ☐
	<hr>**CLOSED CASES: Code reason for
	                        closure**
	1 Aim achieved.
	2 Aims partly achieved.
	3 Aims cannot be effected.
	4 No Priority
	5 Contact not achieved.
	6 Client withdrew.
	7 Client left area. ☐
	8 Client died.
	9 Case transferred.

<u>FOLLOW UP</u> Date for Review Appointment ⬚⬚⬚⬚⬚⬚ Result	

Case Recognition: the Use of Vignettes in Eliciting the Social Work Response

Isobel Freeman

Despite much rhetoric about the development of community care,[1,2,3,4] the development of community based resources for those with health problems has been limited. This is particularly true when considering the area of mental health. Martin,[5] reviewing the development of community mental health services, identified two resource constraints. First, a lack of physical resources such as sheltered housing and day care facilities; and second, the limited extent to which social workers address mental health problems in their day to day casework.

Very little research has been undertaken into mental health social work. Fisher et al.[6] identify the last major study in Britain as being that of Rehin and Martin,[7] which was published in 1968. In their own study Fisher et al. looked in detail at the mental health work being undertaken in three area teams, but before tackling the issue of identifying responses to mental health problems, they were faced with the problem of defining what should be classified as mental health work. They defined as mental health cases, those characterised by impaired social functioning and an impaired mental state - where the impaired social functioning was seen as the result of the impaired mental state. A third of the social workers rejected this definition and some did not cooperate.

In Strathclyde in 1985 a group of members and officers of the Council and of the local health boards was set up to try to identify and promote a more coordinated community-based service for those with mental health problems.[8] As part of their review of existing services they asked the research section for information on how social workers perceived and identified mental health problems.

One method used to do this involved asking social workers how they would respond to three hypothetical referrals. They were based on three real referrals which had been made to the department in the past. The responses to the vignettes provided comparative information on how different social workers perceived and responded to the same referral. Specifically, social workers were asked what indications there were that each of the referrals contained mental health problems.

Responses to hypothetical referrals

Referral no. 1

The first referral involved Jean, a 38 year old personal secretary. She was described as attractive, well groomed, good at her work and popular. The reason
for referral was that her house was in a filthy state, full of old bottles, empty tins,
household and personal waste. The Housing Department had been unsuccessful
in trying to get Jean to tidy up. The referral also stated that Jean's tyrannical
mother, with whom she had lived, had recently died. Jean had refused to see a
social worker.

Those interviewed were asked what steps they would take on receiving this referral.
All appeared to feel that people had the right to live in a mess if they wanted to, providing this was not harming anyone else. However, the response they proposed to
make to the situation varied from worker to worker. Of the thirty-two social workers interviewed, ten said they would refer the case back to the Housing Department and ask them to do more work. One said she would accept the refusal to see
a social worker and do nothing and five said that they would accept the refusal, but
that they would pass the information on to a GP. Thirteen social workers said they
would contact the client and repeat the offer of social work help, but stressed that
if she was reluctant they would not press her. Only three social workers said they
would contact her and take some action, despite the fact that the woman's reluctance made it unlikely that much useful work could be done with this referral.

When asked what indications there were that there was a mental health problem, eleven said there were none, eighteen cited the contradictions in her lifestyle,
two bereavement and one the state of the house. Three said that this type of referral would be given high priority in their team, ten medium priority and nineteen low
priority. Priority was generally seen as low because Jean was single, not harming
anyone, and because she was reluctant to accept help. The following comments concerning priority were made:-

> 'I had a referral which was similar to this. The net result of the referral was that
> nothing was done. I went to see him, but there was no statutory reason for
> involvement. It's a housing management problem.'

> 'It wouldn't be a priority unless eviction was threatened.'

REFERRAL NO. 1

Steps	Team 1	Team 2	Team 3	Total
Contact, but stress that they'd accept refusal	4	5	4	13
Contact and do some work	1		2	3
Accept refusal	1			1
Refer back to housing for more work	6	2	2	10
Refer to GP	2	2	1	5
Refer to home maker	2			

Indications				
None	7	3	1	11
Contradictions	6	6	6	18
Bereavement	1		1	2
House in bad state			1	1

Priority				
High		1	2	3
Medium	1	5	4	10
Low	13	3	3	19

REFERRAL NO. 2

Steps	Team 1	Team 2	Team 3	Total
Talk to couple	14	9	9	32
Ask about hospital social work follow-up	3	3	2	8
Contact hospital		2	1	3
Contact GP		4	1	5
Contact school		1	1	2
Contact Health Visitor		2	1	3
Look at his escapism	1	3	3	7
Look at his drinking/drugs	3	2	3	8
Use a homemaker	6	4	1	11
Look at finance	4	2	1	7
Find community resources	2	1	1	4
Refer to marriage guidance		2		2

Indications				
None	4	1	2	7
Hospital treatment	7		3	10
Depression	6	6	6	18
Drug overdose	6	5	3	14
Escapist drinking			4	4

Priority				
High	8	8	8	24
Medium	5	1	1	7
Low	1			1

Referral no. 2

> The second referral concerned John, a twenty-seven year old married man with two young children who was admitted to hospital after taking an overdose. He had been treated by his GP for depression, had severe marital problems and spent a lot of time in pubs and betting shops, spending a lot of the family's DHSS income. His wife, it was stated, was not a competent housewife, the children always had colds or something wrong with them and, according to John, his wife slept around.

All the social workers interviewed said that they would go and talk to the couple in their home. Most also mentioned several additional steps which they would take. Eight said they would try and find out more about the hospital social work follow-up, some feeling that more should be done by the hospital social workers before transferring the case. Several mentioned the need for liaison between themselves and other professionals, three saying they would liaise with hospital staff, five with the GP, two with the school and three with the health visitor. When discussing John's problems, seven said they would get him to confront his escapism and seven said that they would concentrate on his drinking, four suggesting that they might refer him for specialist advice (either to an Alcohol Information Centre or to an Alcohol Treatment Unit, depending on the resources available in their area). One worker said she would have a look at the drugs he was taking.

Many social workers, when faced with this referral, concentrated on the family's problems rather than on John. Eleven said that they would use a homemaker, seven that they would look at the family's financial problems, four that they would find community resources such as day nurseries or some form of group for the children, two that they would refer the couple to marriage guidance, and one that they would look at the home management. All of the social workers interviewed stressed the need to work with the family as a whole, and they all wanted to talk to the couple together at some point. The extent to which workers emphasised the family's problems varied, but to most social workers, it was clearly central to the work they envisaged doing.

The following comments illustrate this:

> 'John's mental health problems would not be a priority. If this became a case, it would centre on the children.'

> 'I would be more concerned about the family than the man's depression.'

> 'Social workers tend to gravitate towards the children.'

When asked what indications there were that mental health problems existed in the case, seven workers said there were no indications. However, ten felt that the fact John received psychiatric hospital treatment indicated that he had a mental health problem, 18 specifically cited his being treated for depression and 14 felt that his drug overdose indicated a problem. His escapism was cited as an indication by two workers, his drinking by two, and his financial problems by one. Clearly perceptions of what constituted a mental health problem varied. While many workers felt his depression indicated that he had a problem, one worker was more sceptical:

> 'His depression is probably a perfectly normal reaction to the circumstances he is living in.'

Views on priority varied only slightly, twenty-four said high, seven medium and one low. Many workers stated that the fact that there were children involved would lead to the case being given high priority. Some however, said that the priority would not be high unless the children were at risk. Some workers felt that the children's frequent colds were an indication that they were at risk while others viewed them as irrelevant. Of the eight who did not give the case high priority, one stated:

> 'Work with this case would fall into a preventive category and doing preventive work is a luxury in this team where so many of the cases are at crisis point.'

Referral no. 3

The third referral presented for consideration was that of Jackson Curran, a forty-seven year old unemployed man who had been receiving treatment for depression as an in-patient. Over the past twelve years, he had had five periods as an in-patient and his condition was aggravated by heavy drinking and poor physical health. His wife had left him eighteen months previously because of his odd behaviour, drinking and violence. He lived alone in a Council flat and had financial problems. When depressed, he was violent and suicidal and his latest admission was under Section 24 of the Mental Health Act. He was currently detained under Section 26 and was shortly to return home with medication, which was to be supervised by the community psychiatrist nurse. The hospital felt social work help was necessary, particularly in view of his social isolation. The hospital was transferring the case to the area team.

Thirty one of the social workers said they would visit him, one worker said she would not accept the case but would refer it back to the hospital social workers for them to do further work. A variety of additional steps were felt to be appropriate. Liaison was seen as particularly important: nine said they would need to get more information from the hospital and eight planned close liaison with the community psychiatric nurse. Two said they would talk to the GP.

Many of those responding identified direct work they would wish to undertake with Mr Curran. Eighteen said they would identify community resources which would be used to help decrease his social isolation, six suggesting it might be possible to encourage him to be a volunteer helper in some resource. Eighteen said that they would look at his drink problem, thirteen saying they would refer him for advice to the Alcohol Information Centre, A.A. or the Council on Alcoholism; eight said they would try and investigate with him the cause of depression; one said he would look at his violence and nine said that they would try and build up a relationship of trust. Practical help was felt to be appropriate by several workers, twelve saying they would help him budget, eight that they would do a benefits check, eight that they would use a homemaker and one that she would act as an advocate for him.

Many social workers, it appeared, felt they had a lot to offer in this case:

'I would use practical help as a way in. I would like to identify community resources which he could be involved in, although it is difficult to find this type of resource for a man.'

'He may respond well to social work counselling, like this, it may be more appropriate than psychiatric advice.'

'In the past, his involvement with social work has been when he was compulsorily admitted. I would like to build up a relationship with him and show him that social work has other help to offer.'

Other workers were less optimistic about the help they could give:

'It's difficult to know where to start, he doesn't have anything going for him. He is unemployed, his wife has left him, he has no reason to stop drinking. This case would need intensive work and we wouldn't have the time to give it that level of intervention. I would like to try and help him become a volunteer helper somewhere, but there are so many people unemployed that volunteers are not really needed.'

'It's easy to deal with people's drink problems because resources are available. There are no resources for people who just have mental health problems.'

When asked what indications there were that there was a mental health problem, four stated they did not think that there was any complete proof, twenty-two felt the fact that he had been sectioned was sufficient proof itself, eleven mentioned his depression, eight his odd behaviour, five the long term nature of the problem, five his

REFERRAL NO. 3

Steps	Team 1	Team 2	Team 3	Total
Visit him	14	9	8	31
Refer back to hospital			1	1
Check facts with hospital	3	4	2	9
Liaise with CPN	4		4	8
Talk to GP		2		2
Identify community resources	7	6	5	18
Look at drink problem	9	3	6	18
Investigate cause of depression	3	3	2	8
Build up relationship	4		5	9
Help budget	8	4		12
Do benefits check	6	2		8
Use homemaker	6	2		8

Indications				
Long term problem		3	2	5
Odd behaviour	3	2	3	8
Drinking		2	2	4
Depression	1	5	5	11
Sections	12	6	4	22
Suicidal	1	1	3	5
Violence		3	1	4

Priority				
High	2		1	3
Medium	7	4	2	13
Low	5	5	6	16

suicidal tendencies, four his violence, four his drinking, and one his inability to sustain a relationship. There was little agreement on what priority this case would be given in their team, three said high, thirteen medium, and sixteen low. Only one worker referred to the statutory nature of the work. Despite the fact that most social workers felt there was much appropriate work which they could do, the majority felt it unlikely that such a referral would become a case. Most of those who said it would be given low priority said that this was because he was a single male.

'This would not be a high priority and we are only dealing with high priority cases. We only deal with cases which have a childcare element.'

'It would be low priority for social work time, but we might be able to allocate the case to a social worker, but get a homemaker to do most of the work.'

Discussion

From the responses to these three referrals, it is clear that social workers vary in their perception of what constitutes a mental health problem, in what aspects of the referral they identify as requiring to be worked on and in how they envisage themselves responding. Meaningful discussion about what constitutes mental health social work in area teams and the way such work should be developed can only take place if these differing views are identified and addressed. The use of vignettes to stimulate discussion provides one useful way of doing so, and the greatest value of the study reported above is probably methodological.

In relation to substantive issues, the Strathclyde study confirmed Fisher et al.[6] in showing that priority in area teams was clearly given to cases where there was a child care component, and the child care component of any case was usually the aspect of the case on which work centred. The slight variation between the responses given by those from different teams on the work they would undertake suggested workers were, as one would expect, influenced by the resources available to them in their teams. The busier the team, the less likely it was that priority would be given to mental health work. It did appear however that preventive work was often being done on the mental health problems of adults with families, but the problems of single clients had to become severe before any social work help was provided. Martin[5] suggested that the concept of transferability of skills, although widely used, had not been studied much empirically. This remains the case. The responses to these vignettes showed that social workers could identify a function for general social work skills such as counselling, advocacy, practical advice, coordination and liaison. Whether a more specialist approach is also required remains an open question.

References

1. DHSS. *The Development of Community Care Plans for Health and Welfare Services of the Local Authorities in England and Wales 1962-63*. HMSO, London, 1973.

2. DHSS. *Better Services for the Mentally Ill*. HMSO, London, 1975.

3. DHSS and Welsh Office. *Better Services for the Mentally Handicapped*. HMSO, London, 1978.

4. DHSS. *Care in Action. A Handbook of Policies and Priorities for Health and Personal Social Services in England*. HMSO, London, 1981.

5. Martin, F.M. *Between the Acts. Community Mental Health Services 1959-1983*. The Nuffield Provincial Hospitals Trust, 1984.

6. Fisher, M., Sainsbury, E., and Newton, C. *Mental Health Social Work Observed*. George Allen and Unwin, 1984.

7. Rehin, G.R., and Martin, F.M. *Patterns of Performance in Community Care*. Oxford University Press for Nuffield Provincial Hospitals Trust, 1968.

Research Highlights in Social Work

This topical series of books examines areas currently of particular interest to those in social and community work and related fields. Each book draws together a collection of articles on different aspects of the subject under discussion - highlighting relevant research and drawing out implications for policy and practice. The project is under the general direction of Professor Gerard Rochford.

No. 3 Developing Services for the Elderly Second Edition
Edited by Joyce Lishman
and Gordon Horobin
ISBN 1 85091 002 2 hardback
ISBN 1 85091 003 0 paper

No. 4 Social Work Departments as Organisations
Edited by Joyce Lishman
ISBN 1 85302 008 7 paper

No. 5 Social Work with Adult Offenders
Edited by Joyce Lishman
ISBN 0 9505999 4 8 paper

No. 6 Working With Children
Edited by Joyce Lishman
ISBN 1 85302 007 9 paper

No. 7 Collaboration and Conflict: Working with Others
Edited by Joyce Lishman
ISBN 0 9505999 6 4 paper

No. 8 Evaluation 2nd Edition
Edited by Joyce Lishman
ISBN 1 85302 006 0 hardback

No. 9 Social Work in Rural and Urban Areas
Edited by Joyce Lishman
ISBN 0 9505999 8 0 paper

No. 10 Approaches to Addiction
Edited by Joyce Lishman
and Gordon Horobin
ISBN 1 85091 000 6 hardback
ISBN 1 85091 001 4 paper

No. 11 Responding to Mental Illness
Edited by Gordon Horobin
ISBN 1 85091 005 7 paper

No. 12 The Family: Context or Client?
Edited by Gordon Horobin
ISBN 1 85091 026 X paper

No. 13 New Information Technology in Management and Practice
Edited by Gordon Horobin
and Stuart Montgomery
ISBN 1 85091 022 7 hardback

No 14 Why Day Care?
Edited by Gordon Horobin.
ISBN 1 85302 000 1 hardback

No. 15 Sex, Gender and Care Work
Edited by Gordon Horobin
ISBN 1 85302 001 X hardback

No. 16 Living with Mental Handicap: Transitions in the Lives of People with Mental Handicap
Edited by Gordon Horobin and David May
ISBN 1 85302 004 4 hardback

No. 17 Child Care: Monitoring Practice
Edited by Isobel Freeman and
Stuart Montgomery
ISBN 1 85392 005 2 hardback

No. 18 Privatisation
Edited by Richard Parry
ISBN 1 85302 015 X hardback

No. 20 Performance Review In Social Work Agencies
Edited by John Tibbitt and David May
ISBN 1 85302 017 6 hardback

No. 21 Social Work and Disability
ISBN 1 85302 042 7 hardback

No. 22 Social Work Response to Poverty and Deprivation
ISBN 1 85302 043 5 hardback

Case Studies for Practice

Series Editor Philip Seed

The series draws together case material from social research to illuminate and explore vital issues in social work policy and practice. Each volume in the series focuses on valuable material which has been collected in the course of research, especially research into social networks.

HIV and AIDS - A Social Network Approach

Compiled by Roger Gaitley
and edited by Philip Seed
1989 ISBN 1 85302 025 7 paper
Case Studies for Practice 4

A diagnosis of HIV antibody positive - or even the simple fear of it - has profound effects upon the life of the diagnosed person, and the lives of those around them. This book examines the question of how professionals can best care for people whose status touches on so many of society's fears and taboos. Taking a social network approach, it draws on recent case material to explore the lives of people affected - directly or indirectly - by HIV and AIDS.

Victims of Confusion: Case Studies of Elderly Sufferers from Confusion and Dementia

Alyson Leslie
1989 ISBN 1 85302 040 0 paper
Case Studies for Practice 5

The author describes the experiences of a number of elderly sufferers and their carers and considers to what extent their care careers were influenced by the method, timing and source of their referral for service and by the role of the agency to which they were referred. The experience of people in residential respite care is also discussed as well as experiences in local authority and hospital day care settings.

Towards Independent Living: Issues for Different Client Groups

Compiled by Philip Seed
1988 ISBN 1 85302 018 4 paper
Case Studies for Practice 3

'By the aid of clear-cut case studies and copious use of simple network analysis, it highlights decision areas and clarifies decision making.'
- Welfare

'A useful book for both students and qualified practitioners...'   *- General Information, Disabled Living Foundation*

Day Services for People with Severe Handicaps

Compiled by Philip Seed
1988 ISBN 1 85302 013 3 paper
Case Studies for Practice 2

The word 'severe' is used to include those who might be described in technical terms as having 'profound' or 'multiple' handicaps; it is taken to mean people unable to perform most basic daily living tasks without substantial assistance

Day Services for People with Mental Handicaps 2nd Edition

Compiled by Philip Seed
1989 ISBN 1 85302 039 7 paper
Case Studies for Practice 1

The theme running through the cases presented is the extent to which the limits of community care can be and are stretched to provide the services needed by the mentally handicapped and those who care for them.

Introducing Network Analysis in Social Work

Philip Seed

1989 ISBN 1 85302 024 9

For social workers and others in social work practice for use as a guide to the application of a systematic method for understanding and using social networks.

In part one, social network analysis is studied generally; part two deals with specific applications of network analysis. Finally, the role of day care is studied, and procedures suggested for routine reviews using social network analysis.

Social Work Management and Practice: Systems Principles

Sue Ross and Andy Bilson

1989 ISBN 1 85302 022 2 hardback

Much social work intervention is ineffective because it lacks a coherent theoretical basis. Achieving greater effectiveness means more than developing new methods of work, it means looking at the whole basis for social work intervention and developing a theory base which defines how change can usefully be brought about with individual clients and within agencies. This book addresses the question of how this change can be implemented, and suggests some key principles for effective social work within a systems framework. It provides a new explanation for some known and accepted phenomena in social work, particularly in the field of work with young offenders, and challenges the existing theories of how change takes place both within agencies and with individuals.

Which Way Day Care? Analysing Policy and Practice

Penny Youll

1990 ISBN 1 85302 511 9 hardback

Which Way Day Care? is a detailed analysis of the current policy and practice of day care services in the community.

'Share the Care': An Evaluation of a Family-Based Respite Care Service

Kirsten Stalker

1989 ISBN 1 85302 038 9 hardback

The provision of respite care within families is a relatively new development and the *ad hoc* nature of individual schemes has resulted in a great variation in their character; relatively little research has been carried out into the policy and practice of this important development in community care. *'Share the Care'* examines

- the different ways in which respite care schemes operate, focusing in particular on the Share-the-Care service in Lothian;
- the experience of parents of children with learning difficulties as applicants and as consumers of the scheme;
- respite carers: who joins the scheme and why, their perceptions of its rewards and dissatisfactions, and their experience of social work support;
- the less positive effects of separation upon the children themselves;
- families facing an extended wait for respite;
- families who withdraw from the scheme either before or after a carer has been found.

Finally the author draws conclusions about family-based respite schemes, and discusses their implications.

Violence against Social Workers

Dan Norris

1990 ISBN 1 85302 041 9 hardback

Dyslexia: How would I cope?

by Michael Ryden

1989 ISBN 1 85302 026 5 paper

This book draws on the experiences of several people with dyslexia, including the author himself. It is intended to increase awareness of the experience of individuals with dyslexia and to reinforce positive attitudes towards dyslexics in parents, teachers and employers: to give them the necessary knowledge of how a dyslexic is affected, and how to concentrate on their strong points in order to minimize the effects of dyslexia, and find a form of communication that is accessible to everyone concerned.

Dramatherapy with Families and Groups: A Handbook for Social Workers and Therapists
Sue Jennings
1989 ISBN 1 85302 014 1 paper

Dramatherapy is currently established as a methodology and practice for individual and group therapeutic intervention by dramatherapists and other arts therapists. A wide range of professional people integrate a dramatherapeutic approach into their professional frame of reference, including nurses, doctors, social workers, probation officers, psychologists and artists of all kinds.

This book - by one of the leaders in this exciting and relatively new field - is the first to present a working framework for dramatherapists, social workers, family and marital therapists, and others running groups. This framework primarily deals with dramatherapy in the non-clinical setting such as family centres, residential children's homes, social services resources and intermediate treatment centres.

Art Therapy and Dramatherapy: Their Relation and Practice
Sue Jennings and Ase Minde
1989 ISBN 1 85302 027 3

This is the first book to explore the relationship and differences between art therapy and dramatherapy.

During recent years various arts therapies (music, drama, dance, art) have become established in the UK, Europe and the USA in clinical practice and professional training. Each profession has established its own association. What is currently not addressed is how the various arts therapies relate to each other, each, after all, being based on the creative process, while at the same time relating to arts forms generally and to psychotherapy.

The first part of the book explores the theoretical ground on which the arts therapies are based, the history and practice of the two therapies, the relationship between creativity and imagination and therapeutic processes, and the implications for training and for clinical practice of the development of the multi-professional creative team.

The second half of the book describes in detail five major themes that have been developed conjointly in work with students and patients, making use of dominant symbols and mythology. These chapters describe actual method and practice.

Coding the Therapeutic Process: Emblems of Encounter
A Manual for Counsellors and Therapists
With a new Preface by the author
Murray Cox
1988 ISBN 1 85302 029 X paper

'...an interesting attempt to answer the thorny problem of making sequential records of psychotherapy....A convincing plea is made for visual display systems in the place of conventional notes particularly for teaching and research.'
- *British Journal of Psychiatry*

'The notation used has great promise as an extremely helpful conceptual tool for the group therapist in clinical work and research.'
- *American Journal of Psychiatry*

Structuring the Therapeutic Process: Compromise with Chaos
The Therapist's Response to the Individual and the Group
With a new Preface by the author
Murray Cox
1988 ISBN 1 85302 028 1 paper

'...outstanding...derived from unusually diverse experience. *Structuring the Therapeutic Process* is a literate, wise and witty book. It is also eclectic. Dr. Cox has gathered a rich harvest from many sources....There is authenticity and honesty in Dr. Cox's message.' - *American Journal of Psychiatry*

'...rich and thought provoking...a stimulating reflection for those of us who are aware of the unwithering need of organising and structuring again and again our creative doubts. A book highly recommended.'
- *Group Analysis*

Psychogeriatrics: A Practical Handbook

Donald A. Wasylenki, MD, MSc, FRCP (C)
Barry A. Martin, MD, FRCP (C)
Deborah M. Clark, BSW, CSW, MEd
E. Anne Lennox, RN, BSc, MPH
Lynda A. Perry, MSW, CSW
Mary K. Harrison, RN, PhD

1989 ISBN 1 85302 037 0 paper

A practical guide for all professionals who treat mental health problems in the elderly, this comprehensive handbook covers the wide range of problems encountered daily in clinical practice. Topics covered include

- Biological, psychological and sociological changes associated with ageing.
- Common mental disorders in the geriatric population.
- Diagnosis, assessment and management of mental disorders and behavioural problems.
- The contribution of family and community resources to the maintenance of the elderly in the community.

A major difficulty for professionals is to decide what is normal in physical and mental function for an older person. This book provides the means to draw the distinction between normal ageing and pathology and applies this to clinical assessment,

The Science and Practice of Gerontology: A Multidisciplinary Approach

Nancy J. Osgood and Ann H.L. Sontz

1989 ISBN 1 85302 044 3 hardback

The Science and Practice of Gerontology is a reference work for the variety of professionals now engaged in research and practice with the elderly. The collection of articles by experts in each area offers established scholars and practitioners, as well as newcomers to the field of ageing, a wealth of information regarding the discipline of gerontology and the relationship of gerontology to geriatrics.

The reader will find articles on the psychological, social and cultural domains affecting older people, but also those containing general biomedical understandings and practical/clinical applications. The volume presents a series of reviews of past and on-going work in gerontology in those many theoretical and practicing disciplines where this area focus has begun to corner its share of intellectual interests and energies. The authors broadly outline past, present and future issues of theory, research, and practice in their particular area of interest and specialisation in ageing. In combination, the chapters provide a wide-sweeping, multidisciplinary review of a rapidly expanding field of interest.